CH

PRAISE FOR *SELF-CARE DOWN THERE*

"Everyone with a vagina or interested in interacting with a vagina needs to read this book! I just want to buy this book for every woman I know. No, every PERSON I know. This should be required reading on female sexuality, both for those with vaginas and those who are interested in, or love someone with, a vagina."

**—Mary Consolata Namagambe,
founder of She for She Pads**

"The knowledge and wisdom contained in this book is timely as we break into the dawn of a new era in human civilization. We are departing from outdated perspectives on bodies—those of women and all genders—and embracing more enlightened ones. This book is an example of how women around the world are making this shift happen."

**—Halima Al-Hatimy, executive director of
FemCare Community Health Initiative**

SELF-CARE

▼

DOWN

THERE

From Menstrual Cups and Moisturizers
to Body Positivity and Brazilian Wax,
a Guide to Your Vagina's Well-Being

TAQ KAUR BHANDAL

@IMWITHPERIODS

Adams Media
New York   London   Toronto   Sydney   New Delhi

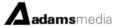

Adams Media
An Imprint of Simon & Schuster, Inc.
57 Littlefield Street
Avon, Massachusetts 02322

First Adams Media trade paperback
edition February 2020

ADAMS MEDIA and colophon are
trademarks of Simon & Schuster.

For information about special
discounts for bulk purchases,
please contact Simon & Schuster
Special Sales at 1-866-506-1949 or
business@simonandschuster.com.

The Simon & Schuster Speakers
Bureau can bring authors to your
live event. For more information or
to book an event contact the Simon
& Schuster Speakers Bureau at
1-866-248-3049 or visit our website
at www.simonspeakers.com.

Interior design by Michelle Kelly
Interior illustrations by Kathy Konkle

Manufactured in the United States
of America

10 9 8 7 6 5 4 3 2 1

Library of Congress Cataloging-in-
Publication Data
Names: Bhandal, Taq Kaur, author.
Title: Self-care down there / Taq
Kaur Bhandal @imwithperiods.
Description: First Adams Media
trade paperback edition. | Avon,
Massachusetts: Adams Media, 2020.
Includes bibliographical references.
Identifiers: LCCN 2019046050 |
ISBN 9781507212363 (pb) | ISBN
9781507212370 (ebook)
Subjects: LCSH: Vagina. | Vagina--
Care and hygiene. | Women--Health
and hygiene.
Classification: LCC RG268 .B43 2020
| DDC 618.1/5--dc23
LC record available at https://lccn
.loc.gov/2019046050

ISBN 978-1-5072-1236-3
ISBN 978-1-5072-1237-0 (ebook)

DEDICATION

To you, reader, for making time for self-care down there. Consider yourself part of the global women and all genders health movement. To really spread the knowledge vibes, a portion of the proceeds from this book goes to charities who promote body literacy across the world.

And to our ancestors whose vaginas got us here in the first place.

CONTENTS

PART 1. GETTING TO KNOW YOUR GARDEN   19

Everything You'll Find Down There

PART 2. SAVVY SELF-CARE   37

Caring for Your Pelvic Area

PART 3. THE WISDOM OF MENSTRUAL CYCLES 83

*All You Need to Know about
Bleeding and Beyond*

PART 4. GETTING WET AND WILD 123

All about Sex and Sexuality

PART 5. THE MODERN-DAY VAGINA 147

Today's Vaginal Trends, Explained

INTRODUCTION

Touch and nourish your body for physical self-care.

Shift your mind-set about your vagina for mental self-care.

*Embrace the quiet and socially abundant times
in your cycle for emotional self-care.*

*Reclaim the wisdom of your vaginal ancestors
for spiritual self-care.*

Throughout *Self-Care Down There*, you'll find a variety of entries that teach you how to prioritize yourself—body, mind, and spirit—by reconnecting with your vagina and pelvic parts, and by allowing you to safely and confidently explore, understand, and nurture yourself...down there.

After all, your body is the home for your self-worth, self-knowledge, and self-affirmation. And doing whatever you can to take care of yourself and your most wondrous parts is something that shouldn't be underestimated.

However, maybe in the past (or even now!) you might have felt that talking about or taking care of your "down there" was taboo. Maybe you felt that it was necessary to treat yourself and your pelvis a certain way due to society's expectations. But today and every day, vaginas are to be celebrated. And whether you choose to speak your empowered truth from the rooftops, quietly nurture yourself in the privacy of your own home, or do something in between, there is no wrong way to practice self-care. You know yourself and your body more than any other person on the earth. And you know which type or types of self-care are going to nourish you the best. So, do what feels right to you. If a particular self-care activity really speaks to you, do it as often as you'd like. If there is one that just doesn't fit well, go ahead and skip it.

So, let's take a look at how you can take the time to indulge in self-care—down there.

A NOTE TO THE READER

I can already tell that you are a magical being. To support your wondrous self, this book shares information about vaginal health, sex (of all kinds), menstrual cycles, and more. The topics are approached from a nonjudgmental perspective so that you feel like your best self when reading. As you know, people of all different genders, sexualities, ethnicities, body types, abilities, religious beliefs, and ages have vaginas. So, self-care down there requires an awareness that your health, body, mind, and spirit are all unique to you and that you are an amazing contribution to the collective.

When you are done reading this book, pass it on to someone you think might need it. I'd also love to hear your thoughts, so send me a comment or DM at imwithperiods on *Instagram* or *Facebook* or find my email contact on the web at https://imwithperiods.com.

PART 1

Getting to Know Your Garden

Everything You'll Find Down There

You are an abundant creature. Paying attention to your body, mind, and spirit sets the tone for how you show up for yourself and the world around you. The seeds of energy laid down when you're nourished will sprout during the low times. This is especially true when it comes to your pelvic parts.

But before you can embrace vaginal self-care, you need to know what parts you have down there, what they do, and how to best take care of them. In this part, using the metaphor of a garden, you'll cultivate information about self-care practices for the parts of your body that doctors call vaginas, ovaries, uterus, cervix, and more.

Remember that even though we're gaining the knowledge in scientific Latin words, every family and community has their own language to talk about self-care down there. You are the child of witches who weren't burned, of mothers who crossed rivers and oceans, and even of families or oppressors who rejected your wild ways. Nurturing a sense of comfort with your chosen and reclaimed words takes time, energy, and money—which you are doing right now. See? You are already many steps into this harvest season, friend.

KNOWING THE GARDEN OF VAGINAL SELF-CARE

Welcome to the garden of vaginal self-care, an outdoor experience that connects human bodies with the earth. Chalkboards, PowerPoint presentations, and uncomfortable desk chairs don't grow here.

To start off, let's acknowledge that each person assigned "female" as their sex at birth has a pretty full patch of land, and it's important to familiarize yourself with these parts right from the beginning. Let's roam through and see how each part connects back to nature on the following list:

- Flower petals: Vulva and vagina
- Sunlight: Clitoris
- Soil: Pelvic floor
- Flower insides, a.k.a. "the yellow part": Cervix
- Compost: Anus, a.k.a. butthole
- Animals and bugs: Urethra, a.k.a. pee hole
- Roots: Uterus
- Plant stalks: Fallopian tubes
- Seeds: Ovaries
- Water: Water you drink and water in your body
- Poison: Vaginal pH
- Bees and pollinators: Hormones
- Leaves: Gut, a.k.a. digestive system
- Weeds: Toxins

Sacred Self-Care

Go outside and find an area of grass, a tree to lean on, and/or dirt pile. Take a few deep breaths and see if you can find the parts of a garden (soil, leaves, etc.) on the previous list outside. Then come back inside to a private place and see if you can find the same parts on and in your own body. Feel your connection with the earth and know that your body is a perfect place.

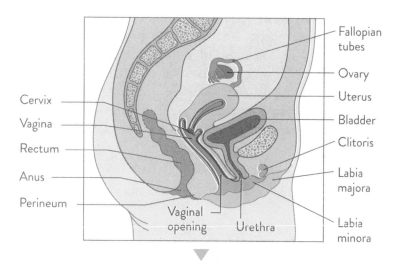

Use this image to locate all of your internal and external pelvic parts. All these parts get put into play because of two tiny X chromosomes, the blueprints for your body. Engage in self-care by knowing all the parts of the pelvic garden and honoring each one.

VULVA AND VAGINA:
THE FLOWER PETALS

Think of the vulva and vagina as the flower petals of your pelvis. The vulva refers to the larger area that includes the urethra, clitoris, and vaginal opening, and it keeps them all protected. The main protective parts are the labia majora and the labia minora, the outer and inner "lips" of the pelvis.

The vagina is like the inner part of the petals that connects to the central parts of plants. It is a fleshy canal that is hidden away yet has so many functions that require an exchange between the inside of your body and the rest of the world. Physically, the vagina allows for menstruation, some sex acts, and even childbirth. Spiritually, it is an energy center that grounds you to the earth.

Traditions from across the world emphasize massage as a way to connect with and heal bodies. You can bring this practice of self-care to your vulva and vagina as well to help you get familiar with your gorgeous body.

Sacred Self-Care

To get started, find a safe space to sit or lie down indoors. If you'd like, you can set up a compact mirror to see your pelvic area; however, a mirror is not required. Once you're comfortable, take your fingers and begin to gently rub the parts of your vulva and vaginal area.

Think back to the garden of vaginal self-care and see if you can touch all the outside bits. What do they feel like? What are you thinking about as you touch them? Is it fun? Is it scary? This practice helps you get familiar with what your beautiful folds and flower petals look and feel like and can relieve tension and engage in self-love.

CLITORIS:
A RAY OF SUNSHINE

The clitoris, the warm sunshine of the pelvic region, is a major source of pleasure for people with vaginas. You live in a world where you are bombarded with negativity in news, facing off with patriarchy daily, and stressed out to the max. It can really wear you down. So, finding pleasure in your body, mind, and spirit can really be a form of radical self-care.

The clitoris wears a hoodie; when touched with affection, it will grow with the love that you give it. Self-care for your clitoris opens up a whole world of dreams, fantasies, and connections. So, give yourself a break from responsibilities, smartphones, and the heaviness of life by embracing your clitoris through self-care.

Sacred Self-Care

Find yourself a safe place to lie down and explore your clit. What is your clitoris's attention span? What kinds of finger motions does it like? How do you avoid nicking it with your nails? Can you even feel it? Are you able to tap into the sunshine? Getting comfortable with your clitoris allows you to connect with one of the many power centers in your body. Not to mention the positive effects that erotic pleasure can have on your sense of well-being!

PELVIC FLOOR: SOIL AND DIRT

What is a pelvic floor, you ask? It's the area from your pubic bone (front) to tailbone (back) that is made up of many layers and types of muscles. The pelvic floor is like the soil in your vaginal garden. It provides strength and nutrients to growing seeds, holds water, keeps all the other parts in place, and generally keeps the garden supported and structured.

Pelvic floor specialists are concerned that one in seven people with vaginas experience some issue with muscles down there that can cause incontinence, frequent visits to the bathroom, chronic pain, pain after childbirth, and/or sexual dysfunction (as defined by you). Are you struggling with a weak pelvic floor? Doing self-care activities like exercising, practicing mindfulness, and stretching can help.

Sacred Self-Care

Kegels are a form of muscle training that involves flexing and relaxing your pelvic floor. To strengthen your pelvic floor, try Kegel exercises throughout the day. They can be done pretty much anywhere—on your commute, at work, at home. There are multiple kinds of Kegels. Some have you get into a tabletop position with your body. Others can be done sitting at your desk chair. Generally, they all do the same thing: strengthen your pelvic floor while taking the time for self-care. See the following illustration and instructions that tell you how to do a basic Kegel exercise and honor your pelvic floor with self-care.

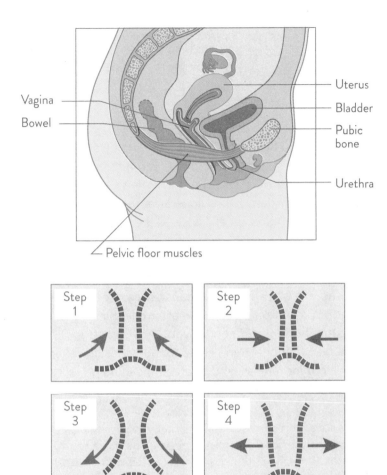

To do a basic Kegel, sit or stand in a comfortable position, then follow these steps. **Step 1:** Slowly squeeze your pelvic floor muscles, so it feels like your vagina is going up an elevator. **Step 2:** Hold the muscles in place for 2–5 seconds. **Step 3:** Slowly release the muscles. **Step 4:** Relax and repeat. When first starting out, you might only be able to do up to 5 repetitions. See if you can continue to practice your Kegels to the point where you can do 3 sets of 10 repetitions.

CERVIX:
THE YELLOW PARTS

Do you know what your cervix looks and feels like? The cervix is a tube-like portal that starts at the top of the vagina and ends up in the uterus, connecting the outside world to the world inside you. It's like the yellow stalky parts of a flower visited by bees and pollinators. The opening of the cervix, or cervical os, is a bustling place where many exchanges take place, like menstrual blood or cervical mucus leaving (more on this later), sperm potentially coming in (depending on your sexual preferences), and harmful toxins being kept out. In the case of childbirth, the cervix is the part of your body that expands and dilates to make space for the baby to come through.

Yet, cervical health is underrated. Usually it's talked about in the context of the human papillomavirus (HPV), which may feel like a scary pest lurking on the plant. But making space to take care of your cervix is important because it's one of the areas of your body where illnesses tend to develop without any symptoms until something drastic happens.

Sacred Self-Care

You can actually get up close and personal with your cervix every day. Next time you take a shower, insert your middle finger into your vagina. Reach until you feel a large bump right in the center—this is the cervix. Search for a small dip at the bottom or side of the bump. This is the cervical opening. If the cervix feels hard like the tip of your nose, then it's closed. If it feels soft like your lips, then it's open for fertilization. Being intimate with your body lets you tune into its rhythms and plan self-care activities accordingly.

URETHRA:
ANIMALS AND BUGS

The urethra is the tube that connects your bladder (where urine collects) to the outside world. It is where your pee comes out. It is pretty tiny, found just above the vaginal hole in the vulva.

The urethra is like the baby animals and bugs of a garden, helping with composting and otherwise chilling out. Like some baby beings, urethras can get sick easily. Urinary tract infections, or UTIs, are one of the most common and unpleasant experiences for the vaginal region. UTIs often happen when something funky gets inside your urethra (like bacteria from little bits of poop from your toilet paper or a new sexual partner). Feeling the uncomfortable itchiness, burning, and constant desire to pee that comes with UTIs can really affect your mental and emotional health.

Sacred Self-Care

Take care of your urethra by creating an affirmation—a statement that helps to manifest goals, dreams, and desires. In the case of vaginal health, repeating an affirmation out loud fires up the brain to think in a particular way. Since the mind and body are intimately connected, the repetition of an affirmation like "My body keeps out beings and toxins that make me sick" or "I love you, body" in a safe place can train your body to think in a body-positive and protective way. While you should always consult your doctor if you think you have a UTI, a urethra-friendly daily affirmation can be a powerful form of preventative self-care.

UTERUS:
THE ROOTS

The uterus is like the roots of a plant. It's a place where every other vaginal garden part connects. The uterus keeps everything else supported and also has its own full-time job as part of menstruation. It even grows, shrinks, and changes position depending on where you are in your menstrual cycle. During periods, the uterus is quite obviously shedding a lot of blood. The rest of the time, it is taking up nutrients and growing the nice fleshy good stuff (including blood) inside it, which keeps the uterus strong and muscular. In the case of pregnancy, the fleshy layer, or endometrium, forms the placenta, which brings nutrients into and waste away from the growing baby/fetus. Notably, during ovulation, the uterus is upright, shining, stretching the whole plant up into the sun. It can also grow large enough to hold a potential baby. Tending to your uterus, the roots of your plant, is a lifelong process.

Sacred Self-Care

The uterus is one of the places in your body that may get a lot of negativity. It's also highly regulated by the rest of the world through synthetic birth control, outdated laws, and more. As a form of self-care, take the time to treat your uterus like your best friend and check in with them. Ask them what struggles they're going through. Are they feeling crampy? In serious pain? Tight? How can you help alleviate these struggles? Also, what are their joys? What positive things happened to them? By adding the uterus to your friend circle, you create space for self-love rather than self-hate.

FALLOPIAN TUBES: THE PLANT STALKS

The fallopian tubes are like the stalks of a plant. They hang out, provide structure, and act as pipes that carry sperm (if it's there). After the seed or egg is released by the ovaries, the end of the tube catches it and keeps it there for about 1 day. This is referred to as ovulation. During ovulation, you might find that you have lots of energy. Maybe you feel like going out with friends, dancing to your favorite playlists, or doing a deep clean of your place.

If you are taking synthetic hormones like the pill, the patch, the hormonal IUD, or any gender-affirming hormones, your body won't be ovulating, so your tubes are just chillin' for the most part. If you have gotten your "tubes tied," then a doctor has surgically gone in to block them off.

Sacred Self-Care

For tubal self-care, try an essential oil massage. Before heading to bed, prepare a massage oil with 10 parts coconut oil and 1 part lavender essential oil. Lavender essential oil has been shown to ease pain and tension in the pelvic area sometimes associated with movement of your tubes. Moreover, abdominal massage is one way to prevent blockage of fallopian tubes. Rub the oil in gentle circular motions just below your belly button. Do not put it in your vagina or on your vulva. Leave the oil on overnight to support lifelong tube health.

OVARIES:
HUMAN SEEDS

The ovaries are two tiny organs in your body that are mostly responsible for every single human life on the earth. They are essentially human seeds and kind of a big deal. For people with vaginas, each almond-shaped organ contains all the eggs needed for a lifetime.

The carrying and release of eggs are your ovaries' part-time jobs (they take time off during menopause). Their other part-time job is to release hormones such as estrogen, progesterone, and testosterone, which connect to all sorts of processes in your body. These include everything from bone development, breast health, nutrient absorption, and baby making for those who want to have bio kids. Since they're responsible for so much work, knowing your ovaries can greatly benefit your well-being across life. What position are your ovaries in? Can you ever feel them doing their jobs?

Sacred Self-Care

If your body is too stressed out, your ovaries can feel it. They will stop ovulating while you are feeling overwhelmed to conserve energy and eggs. One method of calming the body (including ovaries) is to take a bath (yes, baths are the cliché self-care thing to do...but they work!). Draw a warm bath and add 1 cup or 240 grams of Epsom salts. Let the salt dissolve fully, then settle into the water. Soaking in the muscle-relaxing salts, cleansing your vagina with water, and taking this intentional quiet time for self-care lets your ovaries de-stress from a long day (or years) of work.

VAGINAL pH:
A PLEASANT POISON

As you learned in the Vulva and Vagina: The Flower Petals entry in this part, vaginas connect your internal pelvic parts to the environment around you. Vaginas have a certain pH, a measure of acidity in the body. Vaginas have an average pH of 3.8–4.5-ish, which makes the inside of your vagina slightly acidic, like a lemon. You can consider pH the poison in your vaginal garden. You may think of poison as a bad thing, but vaginal pH acts like a poison to keep out anything that might cause you harm.

Your vagina is connected to your brain; they talk to each other about your subconscious experiences, including trauma. When you aren't getting enough sleep, emotional support, or self-care time, your vaginal pH might shift. Vaginal pH can also shift if something new is introduced into your vagina. This shift can cause itchiness, discomfort, and swelling, making you more prone to an overgrowth of unfriendly beings like yeast infections. Fortunately, you can find ways to support a balanced pH down there.

Sacred Self-Care

Take a 5- to 10-minute break to drink a glass or two of water. Water has the scientific name of H_2O, which means that the H, or hydrogen, helps regulate your vaginal pH. Not only does a water break give you time to relax, tune into your body, and breathe, it is also used by your body to keep your vaginal pH at a balanced level. Getting enough water is one of the most important elements (literally) of keeping the bits down there happier and healthier.

HORMONES:
THE POLLINATORS

Hormones are the bees and pollinators of vaginal gardens. They use complex messages, dances, and movements to make sure everything in the body is going through its various cycles (detox, menstrual, sleep, etc.). A little sprinkle of the hormones that scientists call progesterone, estrogen, testosterone, oxytocin, cortisol, and insulin makes your pelvic world turn. And, just as the food systems would collapse without the pollinating help of bees, your vagina and pelvic garden is disrupted by hormone imbalances.

Standard medical practice for the last 50 years has been to prescribe and put people with vaginas on synthetic hormones like the birth control pill, which replace your body's natural hormones with cyborg ones. There can be benefits to having cyborg ovaries, such as pain relief and simplified contraception, but there can also be negative side effects, particularly related to mental health. What you put in your body is your choice. But be sure you're making informed, consensual choices and being aware of your body, mind, and spirit connection.

Sacred Self-Care

Keep a diary for one full menstrual cycle (from one period to the next), writing down observations about your moods, emotions, and actions every day. Tuning into how external factors influence the physical, mental, spiritual, and emotional aspects of your pelvic health brings greater self-awareness. Your menstrual diary can give you signals of where you need to direct your self-care efforts down there.

NAMING
YOUR GARDEN

One of the hardest parts of self-care down there is having the courage to say all the names of your garden parts and express how you're feeling about them out loud. We have all been trained by society to be pretty hesitant about saying words like "vagina." However, by gaining confidence in getting familiar with your pelvic garden verbally, you give it more power and greater visibility in a world that would like your vagina to just be covered up. For example, every language across the world has its own name for the Latin word "vagina," which means "a cover for a sword or a sheath." Of course, the traditional sword is considered the penis, but as you know, the vagina is and always will be so much more than that. In the twenty-first century, the vagina can symbolize self-worth, protection, energy source, and more.

The language you grew up using for your own bodies depends on your geography and your parents' style. But now, it's an important act of self-care to name and develop a stronger relationship with your parts down there.

Sacred Self-Care

Find yourself a piece of paper or journal and write down an empowering name for your vagina. Finding power in names for vaginas strengthens resilience in a world dominated by penises. In a world that is still too often patriarchal, taking ownership over the words you use to discuss your pelvic area is an act of empowerment and resilience. It raises you up and allows you to speak your truth, using words you've chosen yourself—a powerful act of self-care.

KNOWING YOUR BODY, YOUR GARDEN, YOUR CHOICE

For centuries, the vagina has been a site of regulation, control, and oppression—just like the lush land we cultivate and pull strength from. Especially for those who are feeling unsafe or unheard, it may feel like your body and vagina are highly influenced by advertisers, governments, patriarchy, colonialism, capitalism and corporations, sexual and/or romantic partners, chosen family, siblings, friends, and so on. You may sometimes (or even often) feel like you don't have control over what happens with or to your body. But ultimately, what you do with and to your vagina—your personal garden—is *your* choice. Period. No arguments, no debates, no mansplaining allowed. Realizing and embracing this idea is the ultimate act of vaginal self-care that will inform all the other self-care activities throughout this book.

So, dig your hands into the soil, brush your fingertips up against the flower petals, accept the whim of the buzzing bee, and commit to truly knowing yourself—down there.

Sacred Self-Care

Using the knowledge from this book and from your ancestors, make informed choices about what you are doing to your vagina and surrounding area. By educating yourself about the inner and outer workings of your pelvic health, you gain insight on how to prevent low moments and recover after they inevitably happen. Keep up the great work in teaching yourself about self-care down there.

Part 1 Summary

Throughout this part, you explored all the living aspects of a female-assigned pelvis. Each has a distinct role in your body's harvest. From soil to sunlight, pelvic parts such as the clitoris, uterus, and vagina ground you to the earth. Keep in mind the following self-care ideas:

- Get comfortable with naming your pelvic parts. Even the seemingly simple act of being confident in saying "vagina" (or whatever your own chosen word may be), supports your relationship with them.
- Physically explore and experience your garden down there. The idea of inserting your fingers in the vagina to feel your cervix, or looking at your vulva in the mirror might seem terrifying. However, having a sense of your precious parts gives you the confidence to know when everything is going well or when there is a problem.
- Reflect on how each piece is interconnected. While each part of your pelvis has its own name, your vagina, ovaries, uterus, hormones, and the full garden bush work in connection with one another.
- Notice and fine-tune your vaginal self-care mind-set. Self-care down there is not just physical. Take the time to delve into your attitudes and beliefs toward your vagina and surrounding area, with the aim of fostering more pelvic positivity (at least not hate).

PART 2

Savvy Self-Care

Caring for Your Pelvic Area

In today's world, you likely get a lot of information about how to care for your vagina and pelvic region, with advice covering everything from vaginal odor to vaginal tightness, and from pubic hair to pores. There's a lot of troubling advice out there...and a lot of information that stems from messages sent from patriarchal traditions and popular media.

In this part, you'll get familiar with some self-care activities focused around maintenance, skin care routines, and hairstyles for your everyday life. You'll find some health information that will help you keep your down there healthy and the way *you* like it. If you want to pluck, trim, and tidy up your pelvis because that's what makes you feel great, that's beautiful. If you want to reject popular beauty standards and reclaim your pubic hair care, that's perfect too. Just be sure that, no matter which tips you decide to try, you ground your actions in the intention to replenish your cup—not to serve it to others. And if you're scared to change what you're doing down there, it's okay. Shifting your mind-set about your vagina from a negative to positive one is messy, complicated, and possibly super-scary. Rest assured that we are all in it together.

PRACTICING COMPLEMENTARY HEALING

Throughout the modern world, most people access medical doctors and nurses as their main source of healthcare. These healthcare professionals give vitamin shots, prescribe birth control pills, perform uterine surgeries, and order blood tests. However, the biomedical system of healthcare is just one of many healing worldviews. Some diverse healing worldviews for vaginal self-care include Ayurveda and creative English terms for ancestral perspectives. These healing modalities draw on a range of practices like acupuncture, stretches, prayer, heat treatments, and herbal medicines.

You don't have to choose one healing worldview over the other. Rather, you can respectfully gain tools from many complementary healing worldviews with guidance from trained knowledge keepers. By drawing on multiple ways of knowing health, you are honoring ancestral practices that humans have used for self-care down there for hundreds and even thousands of years.

Sacred Self-Care

Not all health practitioners are as open to complementary healing as others. If this is something that's important to you, practice self-care by doing some research on vaginal healthcare providers who align with your values. This can be as simple as asking a neighbor or friend for a suggestion, reading reviews of medical practices online, or going hard-core with a color-coded Excel sheet that compares them by distance, reviews, and credentials.

CREATING A PELVIC
SELF-CARE PANTRY

To support your pelvic well-being, it's important to create a down-there self-care pantry that's ready when you need it. This way, you'll be prepared for your daily preventive practices and for the moments when your vagina surprises you.

Feel free to incorporate modern types of medicine (ibuprofen can be a miracle drug!) and holistic items (like teas and ceremonial objects) that draw on ancestral healing. Your pelvic self-care pantry should be kept in an easily accessible space in your home where it won't get wet or eaten by a furry friend.

Sacred Self-Care

Spend an evening creating your own personal vaginal self-care pantry. Make sure you don't include anything you are allergic to or that has negative interactions with any medicines you are already taking. Notably, do not put essential oils directly anywhere near your vulva or vagina, as they can strongly irritate the skin. Some ideas for your vaginal self-care pantry include:

- Massage oils for yourself, including castor oil and grapeseed oil.
- Caffeine-free herbs for tea, such as chamomile, peppermint, raspberry leaf, nettle, dandelion, cumin, coriander, fennel, or cinnamon. Caffeine is known to increase the intensity of menstrual cramping.
- Ibuprofen.
- Period products: clean cloth, menstrual cup, reusable pads, or disposable tampons and pads.

- Thermometer for checking fertile temperature ranges (more about this in Part 3).
- Birth control methods (if needed).
- Hot water bottle or heat source.
- Ice pack or cold source.
- Journal or paper for drawing or writing, and pen.
- Comfortable shoes for moody power walks.

And any other medicines that you consider essential to your care down there.

GETTING TO KNOW
YOUR VAGINAL SCENTS

Do you know what your vagina smells like? It's absolutely amazing, even if you're not sure of it yet. Vaginal odor is probably one of most stigmatized parts of your body. From scented tampons to eau de toilet, there are all sorts of products out there to get rid of or cover up your natural aroma. The vaginal "hygiene" industry makes about $3 billion a year preying on our insecurities. Sadly, new research shows that the fragrances used in these products are known to cause a range of health issues, from yeast infections to cancer. In light of this news, one significant way you can care for your vagina is to embrace your own unique smell. As part of this practice, you might consider no longer spending money on products that can harm you down there.

Sacred Self-Care

See if you can describe the natural fragrance of your vagina. Does it smell like freshly mowed grass? Like teriyaki sauce perhaps? Or a rich stew? When vaginas are sick, the essence actually changes, resulting in a new smell. This will likely require a trip to a health professional of some kind, but most of the time, you don't need to tend to vaginal scents at all. And you definitely don't need to cover them up or be ashamed of them. Simply enjoy them as you would a rose and flower garden, and sniff away!

EMBRACING VAGINAL SELF-CLEAN MODE

Vaginas have a self-clean mode that gets used every day. As part of this process, each vagina has their own particular brand of discharge that acts like a natural cleaning product. This discharge ensures that the stuff you don't want, like toxins, by-products, old cells, etc., comes out of your vagina, rather than hanging out inside. What this means is that every day you'll probably notice a white or light brown mark on your underwear. This is perfectly normal, and different from cervical mucus, which you will learn about in Part 3.

A hard part of vaginal and pelvic self-care is accepting that vaginal discharge is a beautiful body fluid that sends out signals about what's going on down there. For example, changes in the color and smell of vaginal discharge can also signal that something isn't going well—especially if the discharge looks extra chunky or has tinges of blood in it. It's not something gross; it's a necessary part of having a vagina.

Sacred Self-Care

Practice self-care by taking note of the texture, color, and frequency of your vaginal discharge. While you likely don't have to do anything about it, getting up close and personal with what's coming out of your vagina every day can shift your perspective from thinking discharge is "gross" to thinking it's amazing!

BATHING YOUR BEAUTIFUL
PELVIC PARTS

While you can go days or months letting your bodily smells ferment—which, if this is what you prefer, is absolutely okay—many prefer to take a shower or bath regularly. But not all vaginal cleaning methods are equal.

Whether you like to soak in a bath or prefer a hot shower, how you clean your pelvic parts matters. And the number one rule of taking care of your down there is to not use soap. Seriously, never *ever* put soap in your vagina. It's okay to use externally on pubic hair or your upper thighs, but soap doesn't belong inside of you. Soaps are detergents that mess with the fine balance of vaginal pH that your body is trying to maintain inside and outside; using detergents can cause itchiness, dryness, and other forms of inflammation. Soaps with fragrances and all kinds of added chemicals also introduce unnecessary toxins to the area.

Sacred Self-Care

If taking a shower, run a clean hand or cloth through your vulva. Remove any lint or bits of toilet paper that are left in the crevices. Be very gentle and don't use a cloth that is too scratchy. If you're taking a bath, avoid using any soap or bubble bath, which will irritate your vagina; just let the water do its thing. Taking the time to keep your pelvic region clean is a preventative form of self-care that helps you keep away illnesses and lets you spend a little extra time with your parts down there.

USING OILS
AS MOISTURIZERS

What parts of your body do you moisturize already? Would you consider spending time nourishing your vulva? While it's not widely practiced yet, moisturizing the pelvic area helps with lubrication, reducing dryness, and preventing rashes. It is a physical practice known to support mental, spiritual, and emotional health.

There are endless amounts of products for you to try on your pelvis. Unfortunately, many of them contain harmful chemicals that act as toxins to your body. Consider using a money-saving and earth-friendly organic oil as a moisturizer instead. Basic organic oil favorites are sesame, sweet almond, and coconut. You can find them at your local grocery store and/or small business or online. Just make sure to choose one that you aren't allergic to.

Sacred Self-Care

To moisturize your vagina as a form of self-care, add just 2–3 drops of oil into the palm of your hand. Dab a finger in the oil and apply to the front, middle, and back of your vulva lips. Take 1–2 minutes to lightly spread the oil on all the outside bits—vulva and pubic hair. Don't worry, you don't have to do it in a lotus garden with a waterfall and freshly shaved legs! The best time is right after you take a shower or bath. As you spread the oil, take the time to appreciate your pelvic parts and the role they play in your overall health. They take care of you, so take care of them.

DRESSING
YOUR VAGINA

Did you know that the clothes you wear can affect your vaginal health? It's true! Synthetic fabrics like nylon and polyester don't occur in nature; they're made by humans in labs. They can irritate skin and prevent fresh breezes to pass through, which can lead to ingrown hairs, rashes, swelling, and even folliculitis (a skin infection that develops in hair follicles). Breathable fabrics such as cotton, linen, silk, and fibers that come from plants, animals, and insects are less constricting, and therefore not as foreign to your skin. These natural fibers are more likely to prevent pelvic skin conditions from happening or flaring up.

It's also important to make sure that you're wearing underwear and pants that fit your body. Wear well-fitting (but not tight) clothing to prevent pelvic skin chafing and even UTIs. Forget the sizes on the label: Choose whichever item is comfortable and will make your vagina's life more manageable.

Sacred Self-Care

Keep a spare pair of underwear made of natural fabrics in your purse or backpack. They'll come in handy when your clothes are soaked because it's been raining all day or maybe even when you leaked a little pee while dancing hard. Part of self-care down there is anticipating and being prepared for the "uh-oh" moments.

STRETCHING
FOR SELF-CARE

For millennia, our ancestors have used gentle movements to support blood flow, hormonal regulation, and overall health of the pelvis. That practice is still used today, most popularly in the form of yoga. Yoga poses/stretches or asanas are just one aspect of yoga philosophies from South Asia that are used as a tool for vaginal self-care. They work because movement sequences allow your mind to slow down and focus on the body-spirit connection. Slowing down releases stress, which is known to cause all kinds of pelvic health disturbances. Moreover, the gentle stretches promote blood flow and create space in your pelvis muscles that can keep them feeling pain-free and well nourished. Yoga asanas make a big difference if practiced daily in a safe space like your home.

Sacred Self-Care

For this self-care ritual, get down on the floor and try a yoga asana that stretches your pelvis. You can find options online or you can try the following pose. Don't be nervous about giving yoga a try. Even if you've never tried it before, your body is unique and will tell you when something feels good, or when a movement is too much. And, since you're doing this move at home, there's no pressure to look like anyone else or to worry about what anyone else is thinking. This self-care activity is all about you.

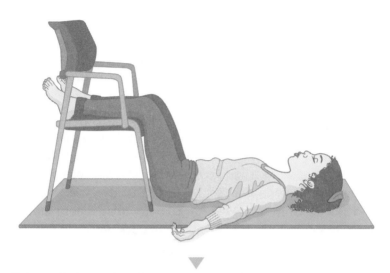

To begin, find a comfortable place to lie down flat on your back, with a chair close by, facing toward you. If you'd like, lay down a yoga mat or blanket. Lift up your legs so that your feet and lower legs are resting on the chair and your knees are bent at a 90-degree angle. Allow your lower back to straighten and the blood to flow down to your pelvic area. Hold this pose for 2–5+ minutes (whatever feels best for your body). Then, slowly bring your legs into your chest like you are hugging them and then rock yourself back up to sitting, or simply roll to one side and slowly sit up. Once you're stable and settled, you can stand up and go about your day.

SHAVING YOUR
PUBIC HAIR

Human beings have pubic hair for a reason. Your bush protects against bacterial infections and keeps your private parts at the right temperature. But while natural pubic hair is back in style, sometimes you may also want to feel smooth and sleek.

There are all sorts of technologies out there that attend to pubic perfectionism, such as hair removal creams, epilators, lasers, hair dyes, tweezers, and good old-fashioned razors. Depending on your skin type and sensitivity, they can either cause your pelvis to feel like it's on fire or feel like a mild massage. Overall, be cautious when using either old or new techniques for hair removal. Find yourself a reputable teacher online or in person who can guide you through the process and/or do it for you. Remember to always use a clean instrument for the job.

Sacred Self-Care

Take a moment to remind yourself that getting particular about pubic hair is for yourself, your pleasure, and your comfort rather than something you have to do to please someone else. So, if you want to shave as an act of self-care, do it! But only do it because you want to, not because it's the "right" thing to do with your body.

TRIMMING
THE BUSHES

Trimming is the safest and probably least expensive of all pubic hair removal. It doesn't cause any irritation and leaves you with enough curls to protect against the outside world, which is an important function of pubic hair. Also, a light trim can make you feel fantastic and can be reminiscent of the chic styles some of our ancestors perfected over the years. And, even better, spending time taking care of and grooming your hair down there (if that's what you're into) can make you feel tidy and pampered.

The basic tools for trimming are a pair of small sharp trimming scissors. To take it to the next level, try using an electric trimmer. Keep your grooming gadgets clean and separate from other items in your bathroom. If possible, wash them with a strong unscented soap and let dry before or after each use. Nothing about strange bacteria festering in an uncleaned pubic comb is going to make you feel replenished and taken care of.

Sacred Self-Care

Take your time when trimming! When ready, use scissors to carefully clip your curls. But prepare for clean-up by trimming over a toilet seat or choosing a spot that's easy to sweep. There will be seemingly endless amounts of tiny hairs that will likely linger for days despite your best efforts to gather them.

WAXING
DOWN THERE

There are so many things to consider when waxing pubic hair. How much will it hurt? How much hair do you want to take off? The sides? The whole bush? Just at the lips? How long is your hair already? Is it more challenging to wax off shorter hair? Can you have sex that day? (You'll probably feel a little raw, so it's best to wait at least one day to have sex with a partner.) When in your menstrual cycle should you do it? (Avoid waxing when you are close to or on your period.)

During a wax, expect to lie down or sit half naked. Then, either you or a salon professional spreads wax over the hair to be removed. In the case of soft wax, you or the professional will press a strip of paper or cloth down over the wax and quickly remove it, along with the hair. Cold wax doesn't require the cloth or paper. Spoiler alert: It will hurt.

If you've never waxed at home before, it's recommended that you do at least one wax with a professional. Not only will you have someone skilled to observe (or wax for you so you can close your eyes), but you can also get tips on which waxes to use at home and techniques for aftercare.

Sacred Self-Care

After pubic hair care, engage in self-care by spraying a pore cleansing toner like clean cold water or alcohol-free witch hazel on the area that was waxed. This will close up your pores and soothe your pelvic area.

DEALING WITH INGROWN HAIRS

Ingrown hairs occur when a shortened piece of hair rolls back onto itself and starts growing into the skin, causing bumps, itchiness, and inflammation. They are the dreaded result of shaving, waxing, plucking, wearing constrictive clothing, and lack of ventilation. Everyone experiences them at least once in their life, if not every time after you practice pubic hair care. You have about ten thousand hair follicles on your pelvic region, so there is lots of room for a pubic hair to go rogue.

If or when you get an ingrown hair, practice patience. Many ingrown hairs will go away on their own over time. In fact, self-removal of ingrown hairs can actually cause infections or scars. Of course, the ideal way to deal with ingrown hairs is to do your best to prevent them as much as humanly possible by prioritizing pelvic self-care.

Sacred Self-Care

To keep ingrown hairs to a minimum, practice self-care and exfoliate regularly. By gently scrubbing away rough skin, you can keep hair growing in the right direction. Once or twice a week helps to prevent and manage ingrown hairs. Choose an exfoliating, unscented product that can be used for the whole body rather than having to buy different items for each area of your skin (unless that's what you are into).

WIPING FROM FRONT TO BACK

Have you ever thought about the direction in which you wipe after you use the restroom? While you may spend a lot of time in the bathroom looking in the mirror at your face, perfectly tying up your hair, or even trying out your best dance moves, taking the time to wipe from the front to back of your vagina can be a huge act of self-care.

For one, it's easier to pick up and feel the texture of cervical mucus when you wipe. You might feel dryness, smoothness, or slipperiness. These sensations give insight into whether you are fertile or not (more about that in Part 3).

Also, when you swipe down, you avoid transferring bacteria from your digestive system into your vagina. When you wipe from back to front along the perineum, which is the skin between vulva and anus, there's a real risk of moving fecal matter into your vagina! The bacteria introduced to your vagina can cause urinary tract infections (UTIs) and other not-so-fun situations.

> **Sacred Self-Care**
>
> The next time you are on the toilet, take a few seconds to really think about your wiping motion. Which way is your toilet paper flowing? Try wiping from front to back. This type of practical self-care may not seem relaxing, but sometimes self-care is about preventing problems from occurring in the first place.

LEAVING DOUCHES IN THE TWENTIETH CENTURY

Douches are not just a curse word for people who have huge egos. The term also refers to liquids applied to "clean" the inside of your vagina and cervix as a form of hygiene. People use douches by spraying water and/or chemicals like vinegar into their vaginal openings to help "clean" out their pelvic parts. If you're douching, practice self-care and stop! As you learned in the Embracing Vaginal Self-Clean Mode entry in this part, vaginas are amazingly self-cleaning. You don't need to spray a cleanser inside yourself to help get yourself clean, and you may even be causing yourself harm.

There are a number of negative consequences of douching. Not only does it disrupt the natural pH balance inside your vagina; it also increases the chance of inflammation in the pelvic area. Inflammation refers to the "invader alert!" reaction in your body when something is going wrong, and it can cause itchiness, redness, swelling, and/or pain.

Sacred Self-Care

For the sake of your pelvic wellness, it's time to say goodbye to douches. Your vagina already has a built-in self-clean program that keeps your insides feeling fresh. So, if you have any douches lingering in your bathroom, throw them out! Then pat yourself on the back for taking such a big step forward for vaginal self-care.

TAKING
BATHROOM BREAKS

In today's fast-paced world, it's easy to always feel like you have to do one. more. thing. before you take a break for yourself. Whether you work in an office, hospital, at home, outside, or elsewhere, research shows that people who prioritize lots of work hours with no breaks have lower levels of pelvic and overall well-being.

Part of the issue is not taking enough bathroom breaks. Yup, you read that right. And it's been proven that people with vaginas have to pee more frequently than those with penises. But taking the time to pee is an important form of self-care that can be easy to ignore. Whether it's because your employer is restricting you or you are under self-imposed pressure to keep working, avoiding emptying your bladder can wreak havoc on your pelvic region. Taking just a quick break to pee when you have to go can prevent UTIs, pelvic pain, and constipation.

Sacred Self-Care

Today, make self-care down there a priority in your life. One way to do this is to take time every hour (or whatever your preferred interval) to take a break and use the bathroom. Not only will you stretch out your body, but you'll keep your bladder happy as well.

STEAMING YOUR VAGINA

Vaginal steaming is an ancestral practice that has been used by menstruators for thousands of years—that's right, thousands! Vaginal steaming involves sitting on a stool with an opening (like a potty chair found at a pharmacy or medical supply store) or squatting over a pot filled with a hot herbal water. Vaginal steaming can help with spotting that occurs after a period by facilitating the shedding of old blood, supports healing from yeast infections, and can even help rejuvenate the vagina after childbirth. The heat and hydrating qualities of the steam are a minimally invasive way of physically supporting the vagina, cervix, and uterus.

Sacred Self-Care

To engage in this form of ancestral self-care, commit to giving vaginal steaming a try by trying out the following steaming directions. If you're a menstruator, steam your vagina for 20–30 minutes 2–5 days leading up to your period and 1–2 days immediately after. Don't steam while you are bleeding; it messes with the contractions that your body is already producing. After childbirth, you can steam every day for 1 month to heal and strengthen your vagina. Postpartum steamers can use gentle herbs, no herbs, or start with cooler steams.

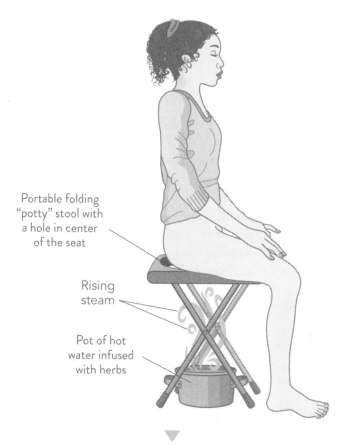

Portable folding "potty" stool with a hole in center of the seat

Rising steam

Pot of hot water infused with herbs

To make your own herbal steam, put 4 cups or 1 liter of water in a small pot. Add 1–2 tablespoons of your favorite herbs (e.g. raspberry leaf, rose, calendula, peppermint, partridgeberry, etc.). Cover the pot and bring it to a boil. Place the pot under the open stool, pour into a clean toilet bowl, or place on a safe surface to squat over. Test to see if it's too hot, but don't burn yourself (watch out for your thighs if you choose the squatting method!). After your steam, drain the water and herbs in some dirt nearby to give it back to the earth or flush it down the toilet.

KEEPING AN EYE ON YOUR FINGERNAILS

Fingernails can be an expression of style, gender identity, and even workload (how often have you put off tending to your fingernails because you feel too busy?). From acrylics to gels to fiberglass, there are all sorts of possibilities for manicures, and many people with vaginas like to keep long nails and even get fingernail extensions.

Some issues can arise when those long fingernails make an appearance inside or near your vaginal opening, which happens when you are pleasuring yourself with your fingertips; checking cervical position by inserting a finger in your vagina; or using period products like tampons or menstrual cups. Keep an eye on your fingernails because they can scratch the vulva and vaginal walls, which can be painful and also open up areas where harmful bacteria can grow and wreak havoc.

Sacred Self-Care

Rather than risking a painful pinch, practice self-care by learning to navigate your vagina with long fingernails. When touching your clitoris, point your nails outward and use the pads of your fingertips. When inserting or taking anything out of your yoni, point your nails inward and keep your movements slow and steady.

SPECULATING ABOUT SPECULUMS

In a typical pelvic exam, your doctor or nurse will ask you to take off your clothing bottoms, lie down on a table, and (most likely) place your feet into a set of stirrups. They'll then lube up a speculum (a metal tool that kind of looks like a duck beak) and ask you if it's okay for them to insert it. Once inserted, the speculum keeps your vagina open enough for them to use a soft, long cotton wand to touch the tip of your cervix for a routine HPV smear and additional STI testing.

During this procedure, the health professional takes off a few cells from your cervix that will then be sent to a lab, viewed under a microscope, and checked for any presence of markers of things that will make you sick ("bad" bacteria, cancer, viruses, etc.).

Many people feel anxious about having healthcare professionals all up in their vaginas, but you can practice self-care by noticing when to leave a situation, calm your nerves, and help you get the down-there medical care you might need.

Sacred Self-Care

Practice self-care by being involved in your pelvic exam as much as possible. Practice saying, "I'm okay with you touching my vulva," or "Let me know when you are just about to insert the speculum. I'd like to be prepared." Take deep breaths and don't be afraid to ask questions or tell them to stop. Then, after the exam, try another self-care ritual by rewarding yourself for making it through the process, like getting a treat on your way home or calling a friend to debrief.

PRACTICING ABDOMINAL MASSAGE

As you learned in Part 1, the pelvic region has a lot going on, a good amount of which happens in the abdomen and upper pelvis. This is where the ovaries hang out and do their thing, where your uterus expands when getting ready for a period, and where your digestive system ends. When your body is struggling to perform the functions of these organs, some people with vaginas will experience fibroids, endometriosis, painful periods, and more that draw their attention to this area.

Fortunately, abdominal self-massage is a self-care practice that can regulate blood flow, encourage lymph drainage, and help eliminate toxins. Such actions can relieve some or all symptoms of pelvic struggles. They can also strengthen your body-mind-spirit connection by offering a tender approach to caring for your abdomen and upper pelvis.

Sacred Self-Care

To practice abdominal massage, choose an oil from your pelvic self-care pantry. Sesame oil or coconut oil are both good options. Then practice the following steps:

1. Find a quiet place to lie down, sit, or stand. If you'd like, remove your shirt or top; but if you're more comfortable keeping your clothing on, that's fine too. However, the oil may stain your clothing, so wear old, comfy clothes as a precaution.

continued

2 Add 1 teaspoon or 5mL of oil into the center of your cupped palms. Then rub it over the insides of your hands to warm it slightly. With the flat part of your hands, rub the oil over your abdomen between your two hip bones and just below your belly button using circular movements. You can go as fast or as slow as you like. Do this between 10 and 12 times to promote the flow of blood and release of toxins.

3 While massaging, you can meditate, think of things that you are grateful for, pray, or just zone out. Push away any negative thoughts about your abdomen or pelvic area. Instead, you can keep a half-smile on your face during the process.

4 Wipe the oil off with a clean cloth afterward. If you would like more support, find a healer trained in abdominal massage who can support you in the process.

SENDING INTENTIONAL BREATH

Every part of the body affects every other part. And every single bit of you, from your brain to your ovaries to those annoying hangnails, is dependent on breathing, which means that tuning into your breath is one way to support your vaginal health.

Notably, many ancestral traditions suggest that the jaw and throat are deeply connected to the pelvic floor. For example, in yogic philosophy, the throat chakra and root chakra (vaginal area) tune into each other. (Note that there are seven main chakras located from the head to the pelvis that act as energy centers for body, mind, and spirit.) Moreover, by sending intentional breath to your pelvis, you can support your health in a holistic way and work to keep yourself from feeling overwhelmed (or breathe your way into and then out of it).

Sacred Self-Care

To engage in a breathing self-care exercise, follow the instructions here:

1 Find a quiet space in which to lie down, sit, or stand.
2 Close your eyes and tune into the rhythm of your breath.
3 When ready, take a deep breath in through your nose, hold for 2–4 seconds, and then release slowly through your mouth. Repeat 3 times.

4 As you breathe in, imagine sending the air down to your root chakra or vaginal area.

5 Know that you are not alone; we are all connected through breath. Feel yourself relaxing or at least slowing down.

DRINKING
ENOUGH WATER

Water is how humans survive on earth. As the Turtle Island (or North American) indigenous community reminds us, "water is life." Yet, in this age of fast-paced lifestyles, endless types of sugary drinks, and drinking water advisories, it can sometimes feel inaccessible.

Making the conscious decision to drink enough water on a daily basis is a powerful act of vaginal self and collective care. With enough water, pelvic skin cells are able to communicate with each other, period pain can decrease, and vaginas will feel extra hydrated. On a deeper level, water is necessary for successful ovulation and for many body, mind, and spiritual processes, such as sacred ceremonies, averting headaches, and preventing every cell in your body from shriveling up.

Sacred Self-Care

Practice pelvic self-care by drinking at least ½ gallon or 2 liters of water a day. It can be tough to remember to keep sipping, but you can make water consumption so easy by following these instructions:

1. Find a new or secondhand ½-gallon or 2-liter glass bottle and fill it with potable water every day.
2. To add some healing properties to the water, bring it to a boil in a pot on the stove and add your favorite blend of herbs (e.g. cumin, mint, coriander, and/or fennel).

3 Keep your water close to you throughout the day and finish it by evening.

4 At the end of the night, thank the water for providing you with the energy you need to survive. Within a few days, you will likely start to see a huge difference in your vaginal and overall health.

UNDERSTANDING VAGINAL FLORA

You may be surprised to learn that you have some bacterial friends living on and in your vagina that you got from the person who gave birth to you (thanks, Mom!). There are more than 250 different strains that make up this little army of vaginal flora. The bacteria eat complex sugars, break them down, and release them as an acid that keeps your vaginal pH steady. If something is off and the bacteria aren't able to eat the sugars, you can experience problems like yeast infections or changes in your vaginal pH, leading to itchiness, redness, inflammation, and pain.

The bacteria also stand guard whenever something new makes its way into your vagina and introduces bacteria from the outside world (like a finger, penis, period product, or toy). Sometimes, everything stays calm and your bacteria figure out a nonviolent agreement with the new entity. Other times, you might get an infection or one of the conditions that doctors call bacterial vaginosis or aerobic vaginitis, which are caused by an imbalance of friendly and unfriendly bacteria. In these cases, it's a full-on war maybe even involving some blood as your body fights back against the intruders. Many of your bacteria will die as part of the fight and a new batch will grow. Fortunately, you can support the work of your vaginal bacteria by eating certain foods.

Sacred Self-Care

Add your favorite fermented food to your meals this week. The friendly bacteria that grows in this food will make its way through your body all the way down there. This vaginal flora will also counteract some of the toxins your vagina is exposed to, like pesticides and herbicides sprayed on plants. Some fermented foods to try as part of this self-care ritual include yogurt, sauerkraut, apple cider vinegar, homemade pickles, kimchi, or achar.

TRYING SEED CYCLING

Estrogen (E) and progesterone (P) are two main hormones that move around your body, pollinating different parts during different phases of the menstrual cycle. In your vagina and pelvic area, they are responsible for supporting your period, keeping your cervix healthy, and regulating your mood. But if your levels of estrogen or progesterone drop during particular times of the menstrual cycle (more on this in Part 3), you can experience fatigue, hair loss, unwanted pimples, delayed or no ovulation, spotting, and more. (See the Resource List for more information.)

The good news is that including certain types of seeds in your diet can promote and encourage the natural rhythms of E and P in your body.

Sacred Self-Care

Practice self-care by giving seed cycling a try for 3 months. You'll need the following items:

- Hand-operated or electric grinder (a cheap coffee grinder will do)
- 2 jars or containers with lids
- 3½ ounces or 100 grams flaxseeds and/or 3½ ounces or 100 grams pumpkin seeds (the E seeds)
- 3½ ounces or 100 grams sunflower seeds and/or 3½ ounces or 100 grams sesame seeds (the P seeds)

To prepare: Add a spoonful of E seeds to the grinder. Grind them up as much as you can. Put the ground seeds into one of the jars. Repeat until all E seeds are done. Do the same with the P seeds. Label both jars and store in a cool, dry space for up to 3 months.

To practice: On the first day of your next period, add 1 tablespoon or 14 grams of E seeds to the same meal (breakfast, lunch, or dinner) every day for 2 weeks. After 2 weeks, switch to the P seeds. Continue this process of switching back and forth for the next 3 months. You'll likely have to restock seeds during the process. Notice and enjoy the benefits of supporting your hormonal health including a boost in mood, a steady menstrual cycle length, and higher energy levels.

HOSTING PELVIC HERBAL TEA PARTIES

Herbs have been essential to self-care down there for thousands of years. They create an intimate connection with land and water to support body-mind-spirit. The hot beverage industry is dominated by caffeinated coffee and tea, but research shows that drinking too much caffeine can cause heavy periods, serious period pain, and even change vaginal pH. Fortunately, herbal teas make a great replacement for caffeinated beverages, and even if you're totally hooked on caffeine, you can still benefit from drinking herbal teas throughout the day.

You can buy herbal teas from your grocery store or at a market; order them online; borrow from a neighbor; or forage with an herbal teacher and learn how to gather your own flowers, leaves, and roots from your own garden. Check the properties of these herbs online or with a healthcare provider to make sure that you aren't drinking something you are allergic to or that won't interact well with other medications, especially if you are pregnant or trying to conceive.

Sacred Self-Care

To make your herbal tea experience a true act of self-care, spend an evening preparing an herbal tea blend for your pelvis. Simply follow these instructions:

1 Start with one or two gentle dry or fresh herbs like chamomile (calm), grated ginger (pain relief), peppermint (energize), cumin (strengthen), and/or nettle (tonic).

2   If using dried herbs, add 1 tablespoon of each to a jar with a lid and mix together by lightly shaking.

3   If using fresh, add 1 teaspoon or 4 grams of each. To brew, add 1 tablespoon or 14 grams of your herb mixture to a large glass jar.

4   Pour 1–3 cups of boiling water into the jar (depending on the size) and let it sit with the lid off for about 30 minutes.

5   Once the herbs have infused into the water, strain out the solids and discard. Then enjoy the tea every day.

EATING VEGGIES
AND FRUITS

Another name for self-care is nourishment, where you give yourself the nutrients you need to not only survive but thrive. How and what you eat can make a big difference to your pelvic well-being. Food is fuel for hormone production, vaginal lubrication, ovulation, and more. So, it's important to prioritize getting all the necessary natural vitamins and minerals that your vagina and pelvis need to function. This is particularly challenging in the modern world when our food is so different than what our ancestors used to eat.

Pretty much all scientists, healers, and grandparents will say that vegetables and fruits should make up about 50 percent of the food you eat; fortunately, you can use certain ones to increase your vaginal health.

Sacred Self-Care

To support your own self-care down there, add the following fruits and veggies to your diet (in consultation with your own preferences and self-knowledge):

- Tart berries like blueberries, cranberries, and blackberries, to help prevent UTIs and clear out toxins.
- Sweet potatoes and oranges to help regulate iron levels.
- Broccoli to help metabolize estrogen.
- Garlic to help with regulating blood flow.

KNOWING THE ORGANIC VAGINA

You know that fruits and vegetables are powerful foods that can help you maintain or achieve vaginal health, but some types of produce aren't as healthy as they may seem.

Unfortunately, modern food systems make use of a number of pesticides that can actually cause harm to your body. In fact, every year, the US-based Environmental Working Group publishes a list of the "dirty dozen" produce items that contain the highest traces of toxic pesticides. For the last 3 years, the following fruits and veggies have made a regular appearance on this list:

- apples
- celery
- potatoes
- spinach
- strawberries
- tomatoes

The vagina and its surrounding area are particularly sensitive to the effects of these toxins. They can cause painful periods, heavy bleeding, or bacterial vaginosis. Fortunately, you have options: You can buy organic fruits and vegetables (especially those included on the dirty dozen list), or you can tap into existing medicinal foods that are affordable and easy to incorporate into your meals.

Sacred Self-Care

Add a splash of organic apple cider vinegar, organic rice vinegar, or any organic vinegar of your choice to your meals. You can add them to a salad dressing or splash over some cooked veggies. New research shows that the compounds found in vinegar can counteract some of the toxins found in pesticides. So, even if you're not eating a totally organic diet, you can still reap the benefits of these organic vinegars...and enjoy the fruits and veggies that find their way onto your table.

UNDERSTANDING THE ISSUE WITH MODERN GRAINS

Wheat. The cunning grass that moved humans from the stimulating life of hunter-gatherers to the stationary life of farmers who had to live next to their fields. It's hard to deny that the cultivation of wheat and grains (like rice) entirely transformed our species.

Unfortunately, when it comes to pelvic well-being, modern wheat is responsible for a host of issues, ranging from generalized vaginal pain to overgrown yeast infections. Compared to the cultivation of nutrient-dense ancient grains of times past, modern wheat is often grown with lots of herbicides and pesticides, bleached, and stripped of much of its fibrous qualities. Many holistic reproductive health practitioners point to modifications made to wheat over the years as the cause of conditions like painful periods and even hot flashes.

Sacred Self-Care

Prioritize your pelvic health by choosing your wheat and grains with care. When possible, soak them overnight, eat fermented ones like sourdough, injera, and dosas, and/or heat grains at low temperatures so that they can start to break down. By favoring slow-cooked grains in your diet, you can ensure that your vagina and its surrounding area absorbs all the yummy nutrients in your food.

EATING NONHUMAN ANIMALS

Since our first days, people have been eating a mix of animal and plant foods. Current research shows that having some animal fat as part of your diet can greatly benefit your health down there. In particular, the active forms of vitamins like B_{12}, D, and A are only found in animal foods. These three essential nutrients are required for pelvic processes like ovulation, healthy periods, hormone production, detox, building up pelvic bones, mental health wellness, and iron production. Note that you only need to be eating meat or seafood once a week in order to see the full benefits. If you choose not to eat meat or animal foods like dairy or eggs for any reason, consider supplementing your vegan and/or vegetarian diet with added vitamins to "beef up" your nutritional stores. While they don't have the full effect of vitamins naturally found in meat, vitamins can satisfy some nutritional deficiencies.

Sacred Self-Care

Spend 2–5 minutes in active thinking mode. Close your eyes and reflect on your relationship with nonhuman animals. Do you eat meat or fish? If so, what kinds? Where do the animals come from? How many times per week do you eat them? Do you thank them or engage in a ceremony before eating? If you don't eat meat, what kinds of fats or supplements are you eating to support your pelvic well-being? By taking the time to examine why you are or are not eating animal products, you can make informed decisions about your pelvic health, which is a form of self-care.

RECOGNIZING FOOD AS FUEL

Eating well can sometimes feel like it's all about cutting out certain foods. Indeed, mainstream diet and fitness messages tend to be exclusive rather than inclusive, perhaps leaving you with a warped idea about one of the most important self-care activities you do in your daily life. At the same time, there are so many factors that keep you from spending enough time replenishing your fuel tanks. You might scarf down meals as fast as you can between checking off the items on your to-do list; feel too busy to cook; and/or even develop disordered eating patterns.

It's important to realize that, for your vagina and surrounding area, food is fuel. It can keep everything happy, lubricated, and itch-free down there. Moreover, certain foods can provide comfort during your periods or during those pelvic health moments when you just need to eat some chocolate. Honestly, giving your body, mind, and spirit the nourishment they need to survive is probably the most important step you can take toward honoring and respecting yourself.

Sacred Self-Care

Whenever you stop to eat, take the time to think of a positive message for the food you are about to consume and thank it for fueling your pelvic parts and the rest of you. Opt for something simple, like "Thank you plants, animals, and bacteria," or come up with a more elaborate ceremony. This practice recognizes and affirms the connection between your body, pelvic health, and the beings that are making it all happen.

KNOWING YOUR
VAGINAL ANCESTORS

You have more than 10,000 years of vaginal health knowledge coursing (literally, flowing) through your blood. All your ancestors had unique ways of taking care of their vaginas. In order for communities to grow, reproductive parts obviously played a critical role. Even today, vaginal healthcare is practiced in unique ways from the Global North/West, to the Middle World, to the Global South/East and all the Pacific Islands.

Many of your ancestors related to their vagina through religious practices, which helped situate them in relation to land, water, the cosmos, and the spiritual world. Religious texts, scriptures, ceremonies, and stories also give us insight into how previous generations related to their vaginas. Whether you pray to a god, goddess, goddexx, or not, spirituality can play a significant role in your vaginal and pelvic well-being. By building up a spiritual practice that aligns with your own values, you can connect the physiological processes of ovulation, menstruation, and more to the universe and the divine around you.

For vaginal wellness, practice self-care by working to balance your ancestral knowledge with modern medicine and your own belief system. Take power from the past, but make sure you're doing what's best for you.

Sacred Self-Care

In a quiet space and seated in a comfortable position, take 10–15 minutes to consider the following questions, as they apply to you: "Where are my biological vagina ancestors from?" "What oral traditions and beliefs surrounding my pelvis have been passed down through generations?"

By being open about where your vaginal self-care practices and attitudes come from, you learn to treat them with respect, love, and an understanding of who has kept these practices going through the generations. However, if you don't want to always align with your ancestral history, ask yourself, "What am I taking from these teachings and what am I ready to let go?"

LEARNING THE STORY OF THE SECOND ARROW

There is a well-known teaching in Buddhism known as the parable of the second arrow. Imagine yourself struck by an arrow right in the middle of your pelvis. Is it painful? Now picture taking a bow and shooting yourself again close to your vagina with a second arrow. Is it even more painful? In sharing this story, the Buddha points to the notion that everyone finds themselves hit by the first arrow, but the second one is optional and often self-imposed.

In the case of vaginal wellness and self-care, this means accepting the capacities of the body you are living in. You will face privileges, oppressions, big moments, and pain. How you react to and grow from these experiences can determine your happiness and suffering.

Sacred Self-Care

Take 2–3 minutes every morning to cultivate a growth mind-set rather than a fixed one. No matter what health situation your vagina and pelvis are in, or what they look like, know that you have the capacity to nourish them as they are, or to imagine fertile futures (with or without kids). Rather than shooting yourself with a second arrow, you can train your mind to deflect it.

Part 2 Summary

In this part of the book, you learned that a big step for pelvic self-care is taking action. You uncovered rituals, practices, and maintenance techniques for your vagina and surrounding area. Some self-care ideas to keep in mind include:

- Create a pelvic self-care pantry. Gather all the medicines, comforting items, and care products you need for down-there care in one place. Your pelvic pantry can include period products like menstrual cups, period underwear, pads, and tampons. You can also include tea blends, hot or cold packs, and abdominal massage oils.
- Keep an eye on your wetness. The various liquids coming out of your vagina tell you a lot about what's going in your body. Cervical mucus and blood show signs of fertility. Vaginal discharge gives insight into your detox system. Arousal fluid or your natural lube lets you know that you are feeling super-sexy.
- Bring movement and breath work to your pelvis. For everyday care, use these tools to support your pelvic well-being: massage, stretching, meditation, and breathing exercises.

- Consume foods that support your self-care down there. The plants, animals, bacteria, etc. that you consume fuel your pelvic processes. Without enough nutrients, immune-boosting goods, or water, your health down there can go downhill very quickly. Remember to slow cook grains; eat fresh, colorful fruits and veggies; and use seed cycling to boost your pelvic wellness.

PART 3

The Wisdom of Menstrual Cycles
All You Need to Know about Bleeding and Beyond

Periods are powerful. Flowing hormones; shedding rich, fleshy blood; and taking emotional journeys keep your soul fluctuating and agile. Menstrual cycles, from menarche to menopause, signify new beginnings, health, and detoxification. That's right, periods have a higher purpose beyond just fertility and pregnancy.

The menstrual cycle is considered the fifth vital sign by leaders in the pelvic health movement (the other four are blood pressure, heart rate, body temperature, and breath). The cycle gives insight into when you need to prioritize certain forms of self-care by mirroring the earthly seasons of winter, spring, summer, and autumn. By reflecting the earth back to you the wisdom of the menstrual cycles has driven networks of love, resilience, hard work, and pleasure since time immemorial by keeping individuals and communities in cyclical balance. At the same time, periods and cycles can be painful. Indeed, you may connect them to physical exhaustion, worrisome leaks, and social isolation. Today, there is still a lot of stigma and struggle experienced by menstruators.

In this part, you'll delve into the four seasons of periods and cycles, and affirm that not everyone's cycle and period are the same. In fact, they are all unique! So, let these entries take you on a journey of self-care from first period to fertility to menopause and everything in between.

CYCLING THROUGH
THE SEASONS

As you know, all bodies are an abundant garden, and Parent Nature has a built-in cycle inside all of us. Just like every other part of the natural world, humans live cyclically; for people with vaginas, periods and menstrual cycles are a built-in way to organize your life. Your body is also a source of wisdom that can tell you a lot about your energy levels, moods, desires, nutrition, and stress by flowing through a recognizable pattern every time. Your pelvis sends out signals that you can see, feel, touch, smell, hear, and sense daily.

Let's use the metaphor of the four seasons to tap into this wisdom. These are the four seasons of menstrual cycles and what they symbolize:

- **Winter:** Period days
- **Spring:** Pre-ovulation days
- **Summer:** Ovulation days
- **Autumn:** PMS or premenstrual syndrome days

Keep in mind that the length of each person's full cycle can vary widely, and even fluctuate cycle to cycle and throughout their life. You might have an 18-day cycle if you didn't ovulate, and someone else might have a 50-day cycle if they are going through menarche or menopause. Your cycle is unique to you.

In your next cycle, start paying attention to the full length of your menstrual cycle by noticing and maybe even tracking changes in your energy, sociability, emotions and moods, experiences of pleasure or pain, sexual appetites, and food cravings. Reference the following self-care checklist and/or download the free checklist for cycling through seasons at https://imwithperiods.com to keep track of everything.

Cycling Through the Seasons:
Self-Care Checklist

Winter: Period Days

BODY PROCESSES

- Both estrogen and progesterone levels are low
- Cervix is lower or closed

SELF-CARE STRATEGIES

- ☐ Stay at home with warm food
- ☐ Don't make social commitments (you'll probably end up flaking!)
- ☐ Engage in self-reflection, drink lots of water and herbal teas

Spring: Pre-ovulation Days

BODY PROCESSES

- Lotion-y mucus
- Estrogen level peaks
- Cervix is low or partially closed

SELF-CARE STRATEGIES

- ❑ Name and play with your desires
- ❑ Make to-do lists
- ❑ Socialize

Summer: Ovulation Days

BODY PROCESSES

- Egg white mucus
- Estrogen levels decrease (indicating egg release)
- Cervix is high and open

SELF-CARE STRATEGIES

- ❑ Engage creativity
- ❑ Take a step toward your goals
- ❑ Hang out with friends and/or network
- ❑ Try a fun new activity

Autumn: PMS Days

BODY PROCESSES

- Progesterone level surges
- Cervix is low and closed

SELF-CARE STRATEGIES

- ❑ Start to gear down
- ❑ Treat yourself to get through hard days
- ❑ Declutter and tidy up your space
- ❑ Let go of what no longer works for you

TAKING IN THE WHOLE-LIFE MENSTRUAL CYCLE

Your first cycle as a fresh, bleeding, awkward kid goes on to inform your menstrual well-being later in life. You'll find that you'll switch up pelvic self-care routines and practices with each new phase. The big transition moments in menstrual health are:

- **Birth:** Coming out of your parent's body as a fresh babe.
- **Menarche:** Releasing your first eggs, starting your first period, and beginning cycles.
- **Adulting:** Going through approximately 300 cycles in a row. Your adult life might include pregnancies, pelvic surgeries, spiritual awakenings, and more.
- **Premenopause/Perimenopause:** Channeling the stormy season that signals the beginning of the end of menstrual cycles to prepare for the calmer weather during menopause.
- **Menopause:** Moving into a period when it's time for quiet, slowness, and calm. Ovulation stops and eggs are no longer released.

Sacred Self-Care

One of the most important acts of self-care that you can do, no matter where you are in your menstrual journey, is to get enough sleep every night. Sleep is the period of time when your body works its rejuvenating magic. Getting plenty of restful shut-eye can be enough to allow your cycle to fall into a steady pattern.

CONNECTING VAGINAL MOODS AND HORMONES

Hormone actions change day to day and year by year. Just like bees, hormones visit all parts of your garden and body, influencing and being influenced by your daily actions. The two main hormones are estrogen and progesterone. Estrogen is produced in its peak starting from winter/period to summer/ovulation. Higher levels of estrogen can give your sex drive a boost, lift your energy levels, and start the flow of cervical mucus (the stuff that looks like body lotion on your underwear). Estrogen helps an egg grow and mature before it's released.

After ovulation, estrogen goes down, and then during PMS, progesterone peaks. If your body has all the nutrients and components it needs, your body's high levels of progesterone will help your uterus grow a fleshy layer of endometrium (the uterine lining) to shed, keep your cervix healthy, and prevent huge drops in mood.

Be aware that, if you are taking synthetic hormones, the hormones will artificially place your body into menopause. If or when you come off of the cyborg hormones, your body will slowly learn to cycle naturally again.

Sacred Self-Care

Schedule an appointment with a healthcare provider of your choice. Take care of yourself by talking to them about your hormones and investigate if everything is going smoothly, or if there are any deficiencies or blocks. Then make mindful choices about the best way forward.

EXPLORING CERVICAL MUCUS

Cervical mucus, also called cervical fluid, is different from the discharge your vagina releases during its daily self-cleaning. It lets you know that your body is fertile and has the potential to get pregnant. According to the popular book *Taking Charge of Your Fertility*, there are four types of cervical mucus textures. Cervical mucus appears during the spring and summer seasons of your cycle, a.k.a. the "fertile window," and can have the following textures:

1 Sticky
2 Creamy
3 Egg white or clear
4 Watery

The consistency and color of cervical mucus lets you know what's going on inside. Sticky and creamy mucus means the body is getting ready to ovulate. Egg white and watery means that it's ovulation game time. White to cream-colored mucus is considered normal; yellow can signify infection (or that you are eating lots of turmeric!); and red or brown can mean there might be some blood.

If you've experienced some or all of these, don't worry. Cervical mucus is a totally normal and healthy sign that your body is doing its thing.

Sacred Self-Care

Maybe you think of cervical mucus as gross, weird, or something to be covered up. Practice self-care by thinking of mucus as a gorgeous reminder of your powerful nature. To test your own cervical mucus, fold a piece of toilet paper into a smaller square. Wipe between your vulva lips before and after you use the bathroom. If you are in the fertile period of your cycle (the spring and summer), you will see some mucus on the paper. Pick it up and stretch it between your fingers to notice its consistency. See the entry on Determining Your Fertile Window later in this part for more information on tracking your mucus.

UNDERSTANDING THE MOON
AND YOUR CYCLE

Have you heard that menstrual cycles can match up with the lunar cycle? It's true. The pull of the moon's gravity on water (think rising and falling tides), and the light it reflects impact the natural rhythms of our hormones. This is in part because our bodies are mostly made up of water. Also, back in the day, before people used electricity and smartphones, the darkness of the new moon and brightness of the full moon traveled through our bodies to influence menstruation. As a result, many people with vaginas experienced synchronicity with the moon: bleeding on the new moon, pre-ovulating during the waxing moon, ovulating on the full moon, and experiencing PMS on the waning moon.

Today, cycle lengths can change a lot due to city lights, screen time, and the demands of modern life. However, many menstruators still report this cosmic connection. No matter where you are in your cycle, you can still draw on the power of the moon.

Sacred Self-Care

Next full moon, engage in a ceremony. For this you will need a candle, matches or lighter, and a small piece of paper to write on. Start by sitting on a comfortable spot on the ground. Light the candle and watch the smoke traveling up to the stars and moon. Write down the answer to the following question: Which patterns or habits that affect your menstrual health no longer serve you? When ready, tear up the piece of paper. Imagine that the thing you are ready to let go of transforms and releases with each rip.

EXPERIENCING DIVERSE PERIODS

There are three main body diversities when it comes to experiencing menstrual cycles: endometriosis (or endo), polycystic ovaries syndrome (PCOS), and fibroids.

Endo happens when the tissue that normally grows inside the uterus (called the endometrium) grows outside of the uterus in the pelvic region. Once in the pelvis, the tissue attaches to other pelvic organs causing inflammation, pain, and scarring.

PCOS is a big category of diagnosis that manifests itself in many forms. According to emerging research, people with PCOS experience disturbed ovulation and low levels of progesterone. Some symptoms of PCOS include hair growth where you might not want it, a strong reaction to eating lots of sugar, and painful pimples.

Fibroids are balls of cells that grow on the uterus and surrounding area. Most small fibroids are relatively harmless and naturally shrink away once you reach menopause. However, sometimes they can grow large enough to cause symptoms, such as heavy bleeding and pain.

Thankfully there are thousands of years of ancestral healing strategies and modern, informed, compassionate doctors who are sharing methods to prevent and manage endo, PCOS, and fibroids (see the Resource List).

Sacred Self-Care

If you are navigating endo, PCOS, and/or fibroids, you are a freaking warrior, friend. As one small daily self-care practice, you can prepare a menstrual massage oil. Use the following ingredients to uplift your abdominal massage practice (see the Practicing Abdominal Massage entry in Part 2):

- 4 parts coconut oil
- 4 parts castor oil
- 1 part vitamin E oil

Mix the ingredients together and store in a dark, cool place for up to 2 years. You can make a small batch, or a large one and keep it on hand. These ingredients are known to have restorative properties that support our bodies through menstrual diversities.

USING PADS, LINERS, OR TAMPONS

People with vaginas are usually in their most vulnerable state when they have their periods. Maybe you hang out lying down in various positions, holding your hand over your uterus, and generally wanting to do absolutely nothing. There is a reason that periods are considered the winter season of the menstrual cycles.

Along with caring for your emotional and mental health during periods, you need to figure out how to receive the blood your body uses to detoxify. It's common for people to use pads, tampons, and underwear liners made by big companies. This is, of course, all good, and please use whatever works for you. However, it's important to note that most of these companies aren't very environmentally sustainable and/or feminist. If that bothers you, consider experimenting with and supporting newer period products that can help to change the way society thinks about catching blood in the twenty-first century. Many products are made by local, women- and nonbinary-owned companies that use untreated cotton and fair trade practices.

> **Sacred Self-Care**
>
> Practice vaginal self-care by avoiding any pads, liners, or tampons that have fragrances added to them. Go for the unscented kind. New research shows that the chemicals used to create the smell are actually toxic to your body. You don't want to be harming your precious parts while trying to catch your blood.

CHOOSING CLOTH

Clean cloth, folded and put on underwear was the way that many of our ancestors managed their periods. Today, you can lean into the practices of your elders by using cloth pads or period underwear with a special absorbent lining. The modern versions are easy to wash, include fun patterns, and may even have snaps to keep them from moving around. And they are great for Parent Earth too. Switching to or continuing to use cloth pads or period underwear saves almost 10,000 single-use pads, tampons, and liners per person from ending up in dumps and oceans, which will support the health of many generations to come.

After all, one major aspect of vaginal self-care is shedding assumptions about our periods and parts down there as dirty, and being able to air our bloody laundry! So, if you'd like, practice self-care by giving cloth pads or period underwear a try!

Sacred Self-Care

For your next period, practice self-care by challenging yourself and using a cloth pad or period underwear from a maker close to your home. If you are particularly crafty, you can even make your own. Most makers carry multiple sizes that can fit all flows. To wash, pre-rinse your pad or underwear in the sink and then throw in with your other laundry. You can also wash them by hand. (It's best to follow the maker's instructions.)

You can bring a plastic bag that you've saved from ending up in a landfill or a trendy pouch to carry used cloth pads or underwear when you are out and about. Keep a spare in your purse or backpack. By embracing the practice of sustainable period products, you can let go of the belief that using cloths for periods is somehow filthy or primitive. Instead, it's a way of getting into right relation with the earth, which you need for all forms of self-care and collective-care.

CHOOSING A MENSTRUAL CUP

Menstrual cups are one of the most sustainable options for period products. They are made out of materials like silicone and rubber that are flexible enough to fold and insert into your vagina. Each cup has a bowl-like section that catches blood and a handle on the bottom. There are many benefits of using menstrual cups. Cups will last up to 5 years and are easily transportable. Moreover, cups can hold up to 2 tablespoons or 30mL of blood (most pads and tampons only hold about 1 teaspoon or 5mL), which means you don't need to check and change them as frequently.

Part of the challenge of using menstrual cups is finding one that comfortably fits in your vagina. Choosing a cup can get so serious that you may feel the need to bust open a geometry kit to measure lengths, diameters, and volume. Thankfully, there are awesome people who have done product testing and can take the guesswork (and the math) out of the process.

> ### Sacred Self-Care
>
> If you're interested in trying a menstrual cup, find one that fits your body by taking the quiz at the *Put A Cup In It* website, https://putacupinit.com/quiz. The quiz is available in several languages and offers suggestions for products from all over the world. You will answer questions about your flow, your cervix, whether you experience any incontinence (leaking pee without meaning to), pregnancy, and more.

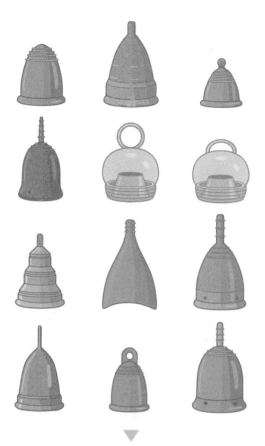

Take a look at all the available menstrual cups out there and choose one that's right for your body. There are wider ones for people who have more space (like people who have given birth vaginally). There are shorter ones for people who have a lower cervix. Some have rings attached to make it easier to pull the cup out. Some have ridges to support vaginas to keep the cup in. Depending on your vagina's history, you can choose the shape that works best for you. Note that sizes can vary among all the different brands.

INSERTING A
MENSTRUAL CUP

When you first see a menstrual cup, you may think, "It's amazing what can fit into our bodies!" or "Oh, heck no...I am *not* trying that out." Getting used to a menstrual cup might take a little while, a few tries, and some hearty laughs. Know that there are millions of menstruators in the world who are using them.

Each vagina has a unique shape, so you may have to test out one or two cups or more to find the right fit. If you followed the Sacred Self-Care tip from the previous entry and took the *Put A Cup In It* quiz, you'll have a good sense of which shape to try first. You also just might not be comfortable with anything in your vagina, which is also totally cool. You do you. If you're curious, check out the following step-by-step instructions for inserting a cup.

Sacred Self-Care
Practice self-care by doing some research before you use a cup for the first time. Watch an online video on how to pinch and put one in. Make sure to really open up your vulva lips. For some people, menstrual cups can be uncomfortable, so listen to what your body is telling you.

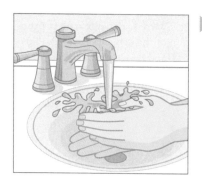

Step 1: Wash your hands and the menstrual cup in warm water. You want the cup to be a little damp to make insertion easier.

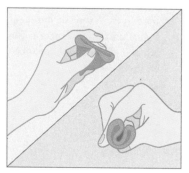

Step 2: Hold the cup in your dominant hand, and use your pointer finger to push the top rim down until the cup folds onto itself. It will look like a closed up flower.

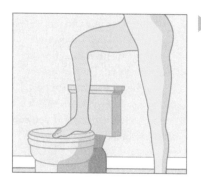

Step 3: Stand with one leg up or with your legs apart.

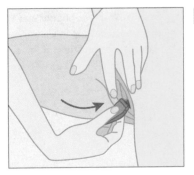

Step 4: Begin to ease the top of the cup into your vulva lips and then into the vagina. You can hold open your lips so you don't snag them on the way in.

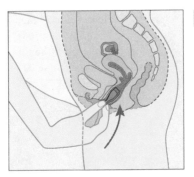

Step 5: Push the cup into your vagina until it feels secure. The tab end of the cup should not be sticking out.

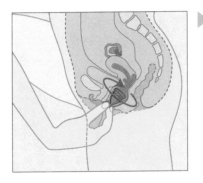

Step 6: Use your fingers to twist the cup slowly and slightly in either direction to create a seal. Then remove your fingers and notice how it feels. You will know that it's comfortably in there if you can barely feel it inside.

REMOVING A
MENSTRUAL CUP

When you first start using a menstrual cup, you may find that the scariest part is getting it out. Being mindful of how you are removing your cup will help so it doesn't feel like you're scraping out the inside of your vagina. The key is to go slow and use your pelvic muscles to push it out. Pull on the stem, tab, or ring at the end of the cup with your thumb and forefinger to facilitate the process. If you are using a menstrual cup for the first time, remove the cup at home so you have lots of space to spread out, relax, and be naked. Hold the cup steady as you pull it out. Once it's out, you can pour the blood into the toilet bowl or, depending on your comfort level, you can pour the blood into a jar of water and use it to fertilize plants.

After you remove the cup, make sure to properly clean and maintain it. This will prevent infections and will also make the cup last longer.

Sacred Self-Care

On the days you are using a menstrual cup and going to be out in public, carry a small well-sealed bottle of water with you to bring into the stall. By being prepared to navigate cleaning a cup in public bathrooms, you can remedy some of the anxiety and worry that comes with this process. When removing your cup in a public bathroom, you have the option of pouring the blood into the toilet, and then use the water from your bottle to rinse the cup clean. Or, while it's not common practice yet, you can support the movement that celebrates period blood and feel comfortable washing out your menstrual cups in a public sink.

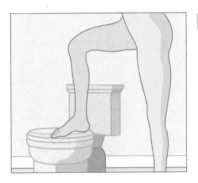

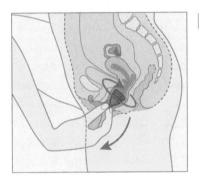

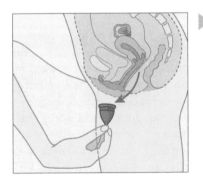

Step 1: Stand with one leg up, or with your legs apart and slightly bent.

Step 2: Insert your pointer finger and thumb into your vagina, pinch the silicone handle or grab onto the ring, and twist to break the seal. Then pull *very* gently.

Step 3: Carefully remove the menstrual cup from your vagina, being cautious not to spill.

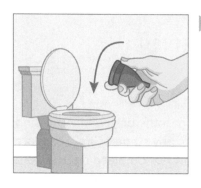

Step 4: Empty the contents of the cup into the toilet.

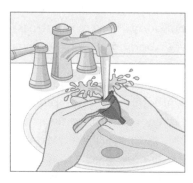

Step 5: Rinse the cup well in hot water with unscented soap, and then wipe cup dry with a soft cloth.

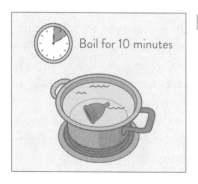

Boil for 10 minutes

Step 6: At the end of your period, boil the cup in water for 10 minutes. It's okay if the cup touches the bottom or sides of the pot. Store in the case that it comes with until your next period.

MISSING YOUR PERIOD

Has your period gone away for months or years? A missing period can be quite concerning at any stage of life. There are a range of reasons why you might not be bleeding. Here are a few of the common ones:

- Your emotions are stored in your body. If you're in a stressful situation for a long time, your body goes into survival mode. It will wait until conditions get safer to ovulate.
- You are taking the pill, the patch, the hormonal IUD, or other synthetic hormones. Synthetic hormones put the body into a state of cyborg menopause, meaning that ovulation doesn't happen. In this case, you'll likely experience a withdrawal bleed once every few weeks that looks and feels like a period, unless your dose of hormones prevents this.
- You are not getting enough fuel and nutrients, like zinc, iodine, and magnesium, all of which are necessary for healthy periods. Without them, your ovaries and organs down there don't have all the pieces in place to ovulate or form a fleshy layer of blood to shed.
- You are pregnant. During pregnancy, progesterone levels stay high, which keeps the uterus lining growing to support the fetus, instead of shedding it.
- You are experiencing natural menopause. Once you reach a certain age (usually 50-plus years), your body has released all its eggs and thus doesn't need to ovulate anymore. No ovulation equals no period.

Sacred Self-Care

Practice self-care by making yourself a nutritious meal this week. Include seasonal vegetables, a dense protein, a small amount of grains, and top with a delicious, fatty sauce. Relish the time you took to give your body the fuel it needs to ovulate and/or keep going.

LOVING YOUR
MENSTRUAL CYCLE

Maybe you've heard the mainstream messaging that people who menstruate or who are menopausal are sick, dysfunctional, moody, and have something wrong with them. Spoiler alert: You are actually magical. Menstrual blood is pretty much the only blood that doesn't come from violence! With that understanding, you can bring forward and foster a positive attitude toward menstrual cycles whether you bleed or not. Of course, as with many things in life, this is harder than it sounds, but know that the wisdom, complexity, and generational healing that comes from menstruating bodies is unparalleled. We are all here because of our ancestors' periods; periods are what will continue to move forward our societies, feminism and all.

So, let's collectively say no to negative period messaging! We are here for each other. We are working together to destigmatize and celebrate periods. After all, our bodies are our first homes.

Sacred Self-Care

Create a vision board for your menstrual cycle. Include images of foods that give you nutrition throughout your cycle, activities and routines you like to do in the different seasons (see the Cycling Through the Seasons entry earlier in this part), and friends and family who support you when you are feeling burned-out or sad. By taking the time to visualize self-care activities for your menstrual cycle, you will always have a reminder to celebrate periods and the practices that support your own and collective pelvic well-being.

DETERMINING YOUR FERTILE WINDOW

Did you know that a person with ovaries, uterus, and vagina is only fertile about 7–10 days of their menstrual cycle? This fertile window, the only time you can get pregnant, corresponds with part of the spring season and all of the summer season of your cycle. The fertility awareness method (FAM) is a modern practice based on ancestral knowledge that helps you track your fertile window.

In a heterosexual intercourse situation, when a penis ejaculates inside a vagina, fertile cervical mucus traps the sperm. The cervix can hold the sperm in little crypts for about 5 days waiting for an egg to release and get fertilized. If the egg releases with no sperm around, then the mucus dries up and the egg usually disintegrates.

No matter who you are, you will feel some changes during your fertile window. Usually people will experience a super-high sex drive, have a lot more energy, and also feel the desire to hang out more with friends. If you are trying to avoid getting pregnant, use condoms, practice alternative sex (no sperm anywhere near your vulva or vagina), and/or abstain from heterosexual intercourse during this time. If you are trying to conceive a pregnancy, this is when you aim to introduce sperm and egg to each other. (Note that if you are taking synthetic hormones, then you likely won't have a fertile window.)

Sacred Self-Care

Managing fertility is a big part of self-care for people assigned female at birth since we are the ones who can get pregnant and make babies. In your next few menstrual cycles, see if you can identify your fertile window by using FAM. Start on the first day of your next period. You can use an app (like Clue, Flo, or Kindara) or pen and paper to track the following:

- **Temperature:** Insert a thermometer in your mouth for 5–10 minutes every morning, then press button and read. See your temperature go from low to high when the season switches from spring to autumn.
- **Cervical Mucus and Periods:** During spring, the body is getting ready to ovulate (or release an egg) and starts releasing fertile cervical mucus—the egg white–textured mucus that you learned about in the Exploring Cervical Mucus entry earlier in this part. Overall, cervical mucus keeps out bacteria and other potentially harmful beings. However, during the fertile window, it changes its structure to allow sperm to easily pass through.
- **Cervical Position:** Stick a clean finger in your vagina and feel for a lump. Be careful with long fingernails. The lump will feel hard like your nose when the cervix is closed and soft like your lips when open (during the summer season or fertile window).

PREVENTING PREGNANCY

One major aspect of self-care in the fertile window involves having safe sex. This can mean gaining consent from partners of all genders (this applies always) and using methods of birth control if your vagina is going to be meeting a penis. In the modern world, there are lots of options for natural birth control or birth control that uses synthetic hormones. They are all pretty effective; it really just depends on whether you use them correctly and what the side effects are. Note that side effects of synthetic birth control can include disruptions to your mental, emotional, spiritual, and physical health. You can make choices about birth control based on your lifestyle, bodies, and ethics. At the same time, it's important for you to make informed choices about what exactly you are putting into your body. The consensual relationship you have with yourself sets the tone for how you relate to others. Note that condoms are the only type of birth control that protects against sexually transmitted infections (STIs).

Sacred Self-Care

Review the birth control options on the following page, where you can find info on natural and synthetic options, as well as one that's somewhere in the middle. Then be sure to practice pelvic self-care by checking out a well-researched website that breaks down your different options for birth control. Be prepared to find conflicting information. Some places to start include https://fertilityfriday.com, http://amandalaird.ca/, www.plannedparenthood.org, and www.cemcor.org.

SYNTHETIC BIRTH CONTROL OPTIONS

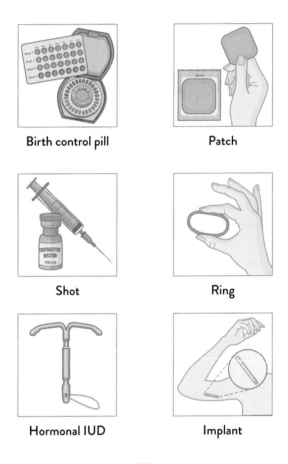

Birth control pill

Patch

Shot

Ring

Hormonal IUD

Implant

These synthetic birth control options are medical interventions that release factory-made hormones that essentially put the body into menopause.

NATURAL BIRTH CONTROL OPTIONS

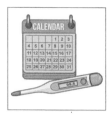

Fertility awareness method

▼

This method tracks the three fertile signs and helps you avoid heterosexual intercourse during the fertile window. Learn more in the Determining Your Fertile Window entry earlier in this part.

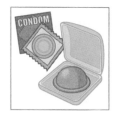

Condoms, a.k.a. barrier methods

▼

Barrier methods provide a cover for a penis, vagina, or a combination that stops sperm from entering into the uterus.

SOMEWHERE IN BETWEEN

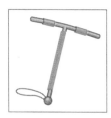

Copper IUD

▼

Inserted by a doctor into the cervix, the copper IUD releases copper ions (or little bits) that float around inside the pelvis in concentrations that are toxic to sperm.

EXPERIENCING PREGNANCY

When sperm meets egg and fertilization happens, a little embryo develops with the potential to grow into a full-on baby. The embryo's home, the uterus, grows a lining called the placenta that will help to transfer nutrients to the baby and remove waste products via the baby's bloodstream. It takes about 9 months (or 3 trimesters) to go from a new embryo to birth, and a lot can happen during this time.

If you or your partner are hoping to have bio kids one day, give yourself at least 3 months to prepare for getting pregnant. During this time, you want to build up your nutrient and energy stores and try to gain as much knowledge as possible about what lies ahead.

Sacred Self-Care

There is a lot of change that happens during pregnancy. Notably, your uterus will grow from the size of an avocado to a watermelon and all the other pelvic organs will move around to create space. If you are trying to conceive or are pregnant, choose one friend whom you trust to the moon and back, and let them know. Pregnancy is an exciting new chapter of life, and it is also when you will need a lot of mental, emotional, spiritual, and physical support, especially with all the changes going down. A friend can help you celebrate the wins and support you through any struggles. Throughout the process, you'll know that you have someone who can witness your story.

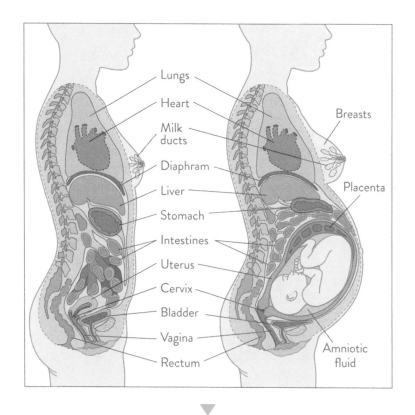

You can see how the body changes during pregnancy in this image. The uterus expands to make space for the growing being, and the organs move around to accommodate it. As you can see, the pelvic parts really showcase their capacities for movement during pregnancy.

PRACTICING POSTPARTUM SELF-CARE

The 3 months after birth, or postpartum, are sort of like the fourth trimester of pregnancy. The pelvis has just run a marathon or fast sprint during labor. This mean that the pelvic muscles, cervix, vagina, and all parts down there need a lot of rest and recovery time. Whether you had a vaginal birth (where your cervix would have expanded so the baby's head could fit through), experienced any complications like vaginal tearing, had a C-section, or experienced more than one of these options, the womb will need time to heal. Your hormones are also in flux and will take time to settle back into the menstrual cycle's seasons. Finally, the mind and spirit have also experienced a huge release; nurture yourself during the fourth trimester by holding a ceremony, having visitors, meditating, reading, or more.

Sacred Self-Care

Support after-birth recovery down there by practicing ancestral rituals that allow you to take the time to rest, heal, and listen to your pelvic parts. These self-care actions can include vaginal steaming, drinking herbal teas, eating nutrient-dense whole foods, meditative walking, and spending time in bed with your new kin. In many traditions, people spent 40 days at home when family members would bring food and gifts. Websites like www.mealtrain.com describe some of the ways that ancestral practices can be brought into the twenty-first century.

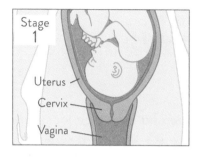

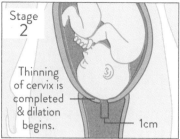

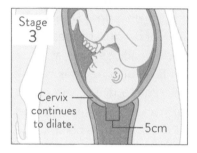

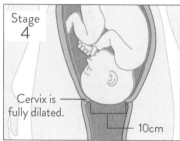

The cervix changes drastically during the process of labor and delivery. Here you can see the process of dilation, the gradual opening of the cervix, and effacement, where the walls of the cervix get thinner. Stage 1: The cervix is neither dilated nor effaced. Stage 2: The cervix measures 1 centimeter and is fully effaced. Stage 3: The cervix now measures 5 centimeters. Stage 4: The cervix measures 10 centimeters and is fully dilated. Can you see why pelvic self-care postpartum is so important?

ENTERING PREMENOPAUSE

Throughout this part, you've learned about periods, fertility, pregnancy, and more. Now it's time to take a look at premenopause or perimenopause, the stage you'll enter once your body releases the last of its eggs. During this stage, which can last up to 10 years, your progesterone level moves up and down in waves, finally settling at a low point. At the same time, estrogen level also decreases. This period of shifting is considered perimenopause. The resulting symptoms can include longer cycles, changes in mood, temperature changes, and more. From a wellness perspective, premenopause is part of the circle of life and can be supported in many ways.

As with any meaningful change in menstruation, a medical doctor may prescribe synthetic hormones, a.k.a. hormone replacement therapy (HRT) to support the changes in your period and cycle during this time. A holistic reproductive health practitioner might ask you if you are managing your alcohol, drug, and/or medicine intake well, if you have passion and purpose in your life, if you are getting enough food as fuel, and if you are drinking enough water.

Sacred Self-Care

For those times when your premenopause symptoms get a little nutty, take some time for pelvic self-care and plan a day at the spa. You can cool off your body, including the uterus, ovaries, and more in the pool. Or, use the steam room or sauna to promote sweating and heat, which can soothe pelvic pain.

SETTLING
INTO MENOPAUSE

The phase after perimenopause is menopause, which can be defined as the absence of menstrual periods for 12 months. In the most basic terms, menopause is the stage of life when your ovaries no longer release eggs, and the levels of natural estrogen and progesterone in your body decrease significantly.

In humans, natural menopause happens organically when we start to reach a certain age, usually between 49 and 52 years of age, but it can vary from person to person. At this time, the ovaries have done their jobs and run out of eggs, and your hormone levels start to shift into low gear. This isn't always a smooth journey, and you can experience bumps and blood along the way.

Additionally, synthetic hormones put your body into a form of menopause. They stop ovulation and the production of natural estrogen and progesterone. If you struggle with endometriosis or PCOS, and/or you want the gender-affirming effects of these drugs, they might be right for you. But if these experiences don't resonate with you, then consider why you are putting your body in menopause and the side effects.

Sacred Self-Care

As you learned before, ovulation helps with bone health, prevents depression, and increases nutrient absorption. So, when the body is in menopause (i.e., when it is not ovulating), your pelvic and other bones are weakened and at risk of fracturing. Support your bone health down there during menopause by eating foods and/or supplements that boost your bone-friendly vitamins—calcium and vitamin D.

Part 3 Summary

In this part, you got to know all four seasons of the menstrual cycle. You learned about birth control, self-care during pregnancy, and the postpartum period, and realized how to take care of yourself during perimenopause. Some self-care ideas to keep in mind include:

- Use menstruation as a metaphor for the environment around you. Periods and cycles connect you to the natural world. By applying the four seasons of the menstrual cycles, you acknowledge the land, water, and beings that keep you alive in the modern world. Moreover, they give you a cyclical way to schedule your work, do household chores, and manage self-care down there.
- Notice the three signs of fertility. Through observation of your mucus, temperature, and cervical position, you are in conversation with your body. It tells your mind and spirit what's going on inside, so you can make informed choices about your pelvic and overall well-being.
- Make choices about your fertility. As a unique sexual being, you can engage in safe sex practices for all genders (more on that in Part 4). For some people with vaginas, this includes avoiding pregnancy, giving birth, caring for your vagina postpartum, and all the chaos in between.

- Respect your menstrual cycle's diverse characteristics. Everyone's menstruation patterns are different. Cycle length can change from person to person, and some people with vaginas have what doctors call PCOS, endometriosis, fibroids, or are experiencing pre/perimenopause. Self-care practices like choosing the right period product and doing abdominal massage and meditation can help you navigate these flows.

PART 4

Getting Wet and Wild

All about Sex and Sexuality

Have you ever lusted after someone? Maybe a friend, classmate, celebrity, or random stranger? Do you ever daydream about a particular person? What is that person's sex or gender? How do you feel about the person physically, mentally, emotionally, and spiritually?

Sexuality is an expression of attraction to oneself or to another human. How each person relates to people on a romantic and sexual level has a lot to do with their own ideas of what they like and their general desired levels of spiciness. We also live in a world where the expectations of society deeply control and regulate the sexuality of women and all genders. At the same time, your desires are driven by your body, mind, and spirit, and fluctuate based on the menstrual seasons, the amount of free time you have, and people's attraction toward you.

Throughout this part of the book, you'll uncover ways to foster an erotic relationship with your own vagina and pelvis. You'll build on and/or unlearn knowledge picked up from media, pornography, and friends. You'll find space to navigate sexual pleasure on your own terms; discover tips on keeping vaginas lubricated for maximum wowza factor and minimal pain; and explore the choices and realities of sexuality. You'll also learn about erotic pleasure through the physical act of sex. Many activists, poets, revolutionaries, and more point to the mental, emotional, and spiritual transformations that come with sexual liberation. When practiced with consent, your unique expression of sexuality is one of the most powerful forms of self-care down there. While sexual pleasure is one significant avenue for sacred connections, you can also tap into the erotic in ways beyond sex acts to think of sexuality in more holistic ways. Let's take a look.

EXPERIENCING SEXUAL PLEASURE WITH YOURSELF

Amid all the noise of daily life that says you need to buy more things or that you aren't sexy enough, self-touch and self-sensuality are forms of daily activism and an integral form of self-care. Indeed, liberation can come from letting go of all the messaging that says bodies with vaginas are things to be managed, covered up, and/or reserved only for reproduction. One way to let go is to actually enjoy having sex with yourself.

The most intimate sexual relationship you can have is with your own body, mind, and spirit. Your "self" is your first home; it connects you to the consciousness of the universe and provides endless sources of pleasure (and pain). The act of taking time for intimate moments and release during solo sex is a sacred ritual.

Sacred Self-Care

Find a safe place to lie down (e.g. your bed) naked or in loose clothes. Using your fingers or a sex toy, decide for yourself what a pleasant self-touch experience feels like to you. The main goal is to have fun, see what turns you on, and break free of taboos that work to control your connection to your vagina, clit, pelvis, and body. Choose the atmosphere that works for you, whether it's quiet or noisy. In safe spaces you can build confidence and familiarity with what turns on your vagina in your own company.

TALKING ABOUT CONSENT

In today's world, negotiating consent is an absolute necessity before engaging in sex with someone else. Consensual sexual acts are beautiful, may lead to a deeper knowing of yourself and a partner, and are also just really good for your overall well-being. However, you likely know through the #MeToo movement and intuition that nonconsensual sex causes trauma, harms self-image, shakes up a person's ability to trust future sexual partners, and temporarily destabilizes the vagina as a powerful center of energy.

Engaging in consensual sex includes asking for consent from a partner, communicating consent, taking no for an answer, raising your own self-awareness, and more. By acknowledging and affirming the fact that your body belongs to you, and that permission is required before someone enters your comfort zone, you are acting as a role model and overall amazing human being.

Sacred Self-Care

Practice taking consent with the next person you touch. Even if it's just a hug to a friend. Ask, "Are you okay with touch?" or "Are you okay with a hug?" and then pause to let them answer before going in for the love! Follow the practice of taking consent when you are engaging in sex and ask your partner to do the same. By always approaching sex through the lens of consent, you encourage healthy boundaries and caring for your parts down there.

RECLAIMING
SEXUAL FANTASIES

The mind is perhaps the most powerful sex toy. You can fantasize during any sex act to keep your mind occupied and your body engaged. Sexual fantasizing is also a healthy way to investigate the types of sex acts that you might be interested in exploring, and your own philosophies of what sex means to you. Moreover, if you want, it can provide you with the space you need to imagine yourself with a partner or an abundance of partners who can share in your erotic pleasures. And, since fantasies are not just about the act of sex but also about the intention behind it, you can, for example, use fantasies to practice taking consent.

Excitingly, this means that fantasies can support the mental, emotional, spiritual, and physical health of your parts down there, your energy center. If you'd like, use fantasy to share in tender love with your partner or partners, and uphold the dignity of people regardless of their gender, sex, sexuality, ethnicity, income level, or ability. When it comes to pelvic self-care, sexual fantasizing definitely ranks among the top ten things to support a sexual revolution, so feel free to join in!

Sacred Self-Care

Think about or write down your ideal fantasy. Sources from steamy romance novels to consensual pornography can be used as inspiration. Who do you picture yourself with? What areas of your pelvis are erotic for you? How are you relating to the people in your fantasy? You can use the answers to these questions to construct, play in, and imagine fantasy upon fantasy for your sexual pleasure.

FIRING UP YOUR EROGENOUS ZONES

Sex scenes in mainstream movies last all of 30 seconds. There's usually the hot make-out scene, followed by some missionary-style hetero thrusting, and then long sighs of relief. The truth is most bodies assigned female at birth need a whole lot more time than half a minute to feel stimulated, pleasured, and juicy. Enter your erogenous zones.

Erogenous zones are places on your body that act as kindling for your sexual fires, and they aren't only centered around the vagina. Common areas of pleasure include nipples, breasts, clitoris, "G-spot" (on the inner wall of your vagina), the neck, and did I mention nipples? The connection between body, mind, and spirit also becomes especially visible during erotic time, adding your brain to the list of erogenous zones. Some less visited areas of your body that may help you get your freak on include hair, toes, fingertips, the creases of your limbs, and more. Erogenous zones can be different person to person, and change over the four seasons of the menstrual cycles. During the summer season, you might want someone to play with your nipples or stroke your clitoris. During autumn you may not want to be touched at all and you may even want to just put on a fuzzy robe and curl into the fetal position with no other people around.

Next time you want to have a little solo sex or sex with a partner, play around with your potential erogenous zones. Some zones might feel better if you are touching them, while others are especially aroused by someone else's hand or mouth. See how many combinations of erotic play with erogenous zones you can try out together. By working consensually with yourself and/or with a partner to explore what turns you on, you can tap into feelings of pleasure that can take you to new levels of sexual satisfaction and self-care.

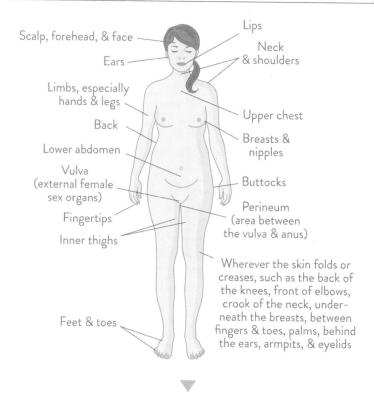

Scalp, forehead, & face

Ears

Limbs, especially hands & legs

Back

Lower abdomen

Vulva (external female sex organs)

Fingertips

Inner thighs

Feet & toes

Lips

Neck & shoulders

Upper chest

Breasts & nipples

Buttocks

Perineum (area between the vulva & anus)

Wherever the skin folds or creases, such as the back of the knees, front of elbows, crook of the neck, underneath the breasts, between fingers & toes, palms, behind the ears, armpits, & eyelids

Take a look at all of the erogenous zones highlighted in this image. You'll notice that erogenous zones can be found anywhere. Your brain can make connections to sensual touch all over your body.

CHOOSING
A LUBE

Finding pleasure in sex requires some careful consideration of partners, location, and lubrication. Not all sex acts require lube. However, if you're planning to fill up your vagina or other spaces with a toy or body part, having a wet, luscious, slippery space can make or break a sexual experience. Using lube allows for smooth entry, keeps your pelvic parts hydrated, and eases some uncertainties about anything going near your vagina. There are three main categories of lubricants on the market. Let's take a look at the pros and cons of each one.

Types of Lube	Pros	Cons
Water-based	Easy to wash off, doesn't stain, most versatile.	Doesn't last as long as other types.
Oil-based	Can just have one natural ingredient, inexpensive, can be used with all sex toys. Liquid or fractionated coconut oil is a sustainable option.	Can degrade latex condoms.
Silicone-based	Lasts a very long time.	Can't be used with silicone toys.

Some types of lube can degrade condoms and sex accessories over time, so be a little cautious about what you use. If you are at risk of unintentional pregnancy, use a water-based lube with condoms during your fertile window. Other than that, enjoy the wonders of silky, sliding, and squirting lube.

Sacred Self-Care

Practice self-care by using lube when engaging in solo or multiple-person intercourse involving a dildo or penis. Spit or saliva is not enough, and sometimes neither is your body's internal wetness, which means that intercourse can cause irritation and pain down there (and not the consensual, sexy kind). And unless you want a very itchy vagina, *avoid* any lotions or gels meant for external use only.

DELVING
INTO DILDOS

Most sex shops call toys that fill the vagina "dildos." Dildos can be inserted in the vagina and/or bum, with consent, to stimulate your internal erogenous zones. There are endless varieties that come in all shapes and sizes.

No matter who your choice of sexual partner is, most of us will try sticking something into our vagina for pleasure. Some for curiosity...and some just by sheer accident.

Avoid using large household items as dildo substitutes. This list includes water bottles, butternut squashes and other gourds, and anything remotely sharp or breakable. Please don't hesitate to explore your body; just keep your vaginal health in mind at all times.

Sacred Self-Care

Choose a dildo with a really solid, long handle that you can hold onto. The handle is the most important safety measure. Start with a dildo that's on the thinner and shorter side; if you find it enjoyable, work your way up in size from there. Using a dildo is not going to be everyone's preferred choice for self-care down there. However, if you're interested, a dildo can stimulate the erotic desires of your vagina without needing a partner. Or a dildo can be used consensually with a partner to help you explore the depth and breadth of your sexual appetite.

EXPANDING YOUR
SEX TOY BOX

Aside from the standard dildo, there are lots of sex toys available that add some spice to your sex life. Depending on the size, sensitivity, and type of excitement that your pelvis and vagina are looking for, you can explore a variety of options. Categories of sex toys by action include vibrators, plugs, sleeves, c-rings, harnesses, pumps, and all the equipment for safe bondage.

Sex toys work by creating friction or stimulation in a particular erogenous zone. They can also direct blood and attention toward a certain area. They can also let you play out the fantasies you've dreamed up. When it comes to self-care, sexual pleasure and orgasms in particular can decrease stress, relieve pain by releasing endorphins, and can even help you sleep better.

Sacred Self-Care

You can support your pelvic self-care by investing in sex toys that help you have a fulfilling sex life. Find an in-person and/or online sex shop that focuses on body-positive messaging for all types of sexualities. They can support you in your journey to experiment with various toys. It's best to find sex toys that are made of earth-friendly, toxin-free materials. Venus Envy, based in Canada (https://venusenvy.ca), and Lelo (www.lelo.com) in the US are popular choices; or you can search for one in your region. Lastly, if you are new to sex toys and don't really know where to start, a small vibrator is usually a good jumping-off point.

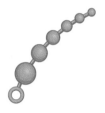

Beads with handles

Vibrators, dildos, and plugs

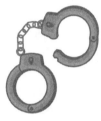

Handcuffs and consensual bondage

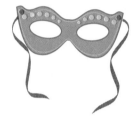

Masks and costumes

As you can see, sex toys give you the option to play out all of your bedroom (or anywhere!) fantasies. As long as you're experimenting with safe, consensual sex play, anything goes!

USING CONDOMS AND COVERS

Cheap and easily accessible rubber latex condoms are one of modern medicine's best inventions. They come in shapes to fit female and male-assigned genitals. They play an important role in protecting vaginas from diseases and from errant male sperm, which can result in unintended pregnancy.

The actual practice of covering up our genitals goes back to our days as Stone Age cave dwellers, but now you have so many options for having safe sex. Condoms now come in diverse materials (e.g. latex, polyurethane, lambskin), sizes, and textures. Even better, many companies are rethinking their ethics of where they source their ingredients and making sure they aren't adding in toxins, which means that you can find a condom that fits both your vagina and your politics!

Negotiating the use of condoms during sex can be a challenge, though. You may not be familiar with how to use a condom, your sexual partner might be opposed to using them, and/or some condom materials may irritate your vagina. However, with the right product that's comfortable for everyone involved, it can be that much easier to have consensual, safe sex.

Sacred Self-Care

No matter what condom type you use, practice self-care by testing out one to two brands, and figuring out which type or types feel the best for your vagina in terms of size and texture. Many condom companies will have tester packs at discounted prices. Some brand recommendations include Glyde, Skyn, and the well-known Trojan.

CHOOSING A
SEX POSITION

For many people, sexual intimacy can be a source of curiosity, release, fun, and a form of self-care down there. For others, it's agonizing. Wherever you are on this spectrum, you can find ways to take up space and decide how you want to move your bodies to experience erotic pleasure. Self-care in sex means tuning into what we want from the experience, and then responding by asking for consent to do it.

While mainstream preconceived ideas of what sex should look and feel like often put penises front and center of many sex positions, people with vaginas can still have mind-blowing sex without them! Much of your sexual pleasure comes from all five senses: touch, sight, taste, smell, and sound. Experimenting with sex positions that use a combination of senses will let you explore your seductive and sensual sides.

Sacred Self-Care

Be patient with yourself and/or a sexual partner. Figuring out what feels good for both or more of you takes time and a sense of safety. Embrace the idea of failing really well at sex, and you'll find yourself laughing, moaning, and orgasming in the right amount of time. And if you're looking for a list of positions that don't get enough play, visit http://teenhealthsource.com/blog/queering-sexual-education/ or www.refinery29.com/en-us/2016/09/124883/kamasutra-sex-positions for ideas.

REDEFINING VIRGINITY

The traditional definition of "losing" one's virginity means opening up the hymen—the thin piece of tissue that partially covers the opening of your vagina. For thousands of years, it's been seen as a rite of passage for women and all genders with vaginas, and has been primarily linked to heterosexual, monogamous marriage.

Fortunately, today you can aim to define what making your sexual debut means to you. Depending on how you want to label it, the idea of no longer being a virgin can mean having sex for the first time with a partner, using a dildo, or even inserting a tampon. Regardless of how you choose to approach it, know that all consensual acts of moving past "virginity" are valid.

Sacred Self-Care

On a piece of paper or in a journal, write down your thoughts about and experience of virginity. Do you consider yourself a virgin? When did that shift for you? How does it feel for you emotionally? What are you looking for in future sexual experiences? What is your definition of virginity?

Don't worry about spelling or making any sense for anyone else. If you don't want anyone else to find your writing, you can burn or rip up the paper after you are done. By taking time to explore your ideas, self-concepts, and experiences of virginity as a form of self-care, you can relieve some of the anxiety, worry, and uncertainty that often come with this very contested term.

TAKING CARE OF
YOUR SEXUALITY

Whom you decide to have sex with can really shape your sexual pleasure. Attraction plays a big part in sexual pleasure; you're way more likely to enjoy a sexual or romantic encounter if you're attracted to the person you're having it with.

Understanding the erotic desires of your own body involves choosing the people you engage with romantically and sexually. Maybe you identify as straight, gay, polyamorous, lesbian, bisexual, queer, asexual, pansexual, and/or more. No matter what label you want to align with, you can work toward supporting your individual and collective pelvic well-being by affirming people's choices in consensual sexual partners and sexual preferences. While where you live may determine how comfortable you are expressing your sexual desires, allowing yourself and each other to live your own truth when it comes to sexual encounters is a powerful type of self-care. Thankfully, with lots of new options for meeting potential partners, you can curate your romantic and sexual experiences to fit your needs and desires.

Sacred Self-Care

Start to have conversations about the types of people you are into. Ask questions like: What are your potential partner's genders? Sexes? What are their opinions on sexuality? What do they do for self-care down there? Whether you choose to keep the questions and answers to yourself, or share them with trusted people around you, having an open dialogue about your sexuality can be healing and transformative.

RETHINKING ORGASMS

As you know, orgasms are a vital tool for your mental, emotional, spiritual, and physical health, but according to research, more than 50 percent of people with vaginas have pretended to cum for any number of reasons. Fortunately, you can increase your chances of orgasming during sex with a partner or with yourself by building trust and honesty with your partners, adding in self-touch and/or vibrators, using the power of fantasy to connect body-mind-spirit, trying out new sex positions, and/or lengthening the amount of time you spend getting your sex on. Of course, it's not totally on you to make this shift. Your sexual partners also need to step up and consider their role in your pleasure.

That said, it's also totally okay to not have an orgasm if you just aren't feeling it or if that's not your goal for a particular experience of sex. Being mindful of your relationship to orgasms and feeling confident in your relationship with them supports your self-care down there.

Sacred Self-Care

Announce a new self-care era of sexual release! Either by yourself or with a partner, take your time to bring yourself to an orgasm by playing with your clit or any other area. Ask your partner to move as much or as little as you want. Draw on your ideal fantasy to keep your mind engaged while you explore the physical pleasures. Let yourself let out a big sigh of relief when it happens! And if it doesn't, don't get discouraged. Just try again another time when you're feeling aroused.

FEELING OUT
YOUR FETISHES

From nipple clamps to candle wax to cuddling with stuffed animals, we all have our own fetish. Can you name yours? You can tap into your vagina's favorite flavor by exploring your sexual curiosities and your relationship with yourself, and by connecting with a like-minded community. And, if you don't have the privilege or consent of acting out your fetish in real life, consensual fantasizing is a powerful tool to test out your tastes.

Sometimes some particular preferences may be difficult to name or accept, especially if they involve the roles of submissive or dominant partners. This relationship might correspond with internalized ideas of being an oppressor or being oppressed, or, you know, just be what you are into. The challenge of kinky sex is being aware of why and how we are doing it, and most importantly, taking consent along the way. And don't forget the lube, which is necessary most of the time.

Sacred Self-Care

Scroll through a list of sex acts and fetishes for all genders or listen to a podcast. The podcast episodes from *Savage Lovecast* (www.savagelovecast.com) are a safe place to start exploring kinky cravings. You can read through the descriptions or listen to parts of the interviews. By getting familiar with and normalizing sexual fetishes and kinks, you can affirm the unique erotic explorations of your pelvic parts.

UNDERSTANDING SEXUAL PAIN

Sex can sometimes (or always, if that's your preference) involve pain.

The good kind of pain is consensual. You may decide to add a little pinch or love tap into your routines with your partner(s) or yourself. Maybe throw in a clamp or two. Or, you know, go full-on *Fifty Shades of Grey*. For some people pleasure can come from the increased blood flow and heightened sensation of consensual pain.

The bad kind of pain can happen by accident, by the nature of our bodies, or through nonconsensual sex. Maybe in the throes of thrusting, a body part or toy ends up where it shouldn't be. In all cases of bad sexual pain, practice self-care by reaching out to a therapist, pelvic floor coach, and/or trusted friend with whom you can share your struggles.

Sacred Self-Care

Find a safe place to lie down and get naked with yourself. Test out where your level of pain tolerance meets being turned on. You can start by gently tugging at or pinching sensitive sexual areas like your nipples or clitoris. Can you focus and send breath to these areas? Are any negative, neutral, or positive images coming up for you? How do you feel about it overall? By gaining a sense of where the line between good and bad pain is for you, you can support your pelvis in its journey to pleasure.

GETTING COMFORTABLE WITH QUEEFING

Do you wonder why your vagina sometimes makes loud noises during sex? Don't worry, it's not a fart! There is no fermentation or smell involved, and it has nothing to do with the whole pizza you might have eaten earlier in the evening. What's happening is something called queefing, which occurs when lots of air gets into your vagina and is then released.

Sometimes vaginas expand if or when you put something in them (e.g. fingers, dildos, or penises), or when you are doing a lot of physical activity. This means that there is more space for air to come in and hang out. Queefing is a totally normal physical reaction, like popping the cork off a carbonated drink bottle. It doesn't mean you are too loose or something is going wrong. Rest assured that when you find yourself letting out a long queef, you are probably doing something that your vagina is into.

Sacred Self-Care

The next time you let out a queef during sex, rather than being horrified or pretending like nothing happened, see if you can think "Ooh, what a gorgeous noise!" Debrief with your partner or yourself about it afterward to see how you can continue to affirm the fact that queefing is a normal and common musical interlude during sex. By reworking your mind-set to view queefing from a positive perspective, you support your vaginal sense of self-esteem.

ABSTAINING FROM SEX

Abstinence means restraining yourself from engaging in an indulgent activity. Are you interested in sex, but making an active choice to not engage in it? When it comes to sex and your vagina, there is a spectrum of choice for abstinence or celibacy. For example, some people have had active sex lives and choose to abstain for personal reasons. Some know that they are addicted and seek out sobriety. Some just aren't interested, and some might be following religious customs.

Abstaining from sex is a decision you have to make for yourself. For example, some people might choose to abstain from all sex acts, including solo sex, and others only from certain sex positions. Overall, abstinence is a practice that can have different boundaries for different people.

Sacred Self-Care

In a comfortable seated position, close your eyes and spend 3–5 minutes practicing meditation. Mindfulness meditation draws on the principles of slowing down, being in the present, and noticing your thought patterns. Not engaging in sex as a personal and/or religious choice can take a lot of willpower for most people. For others, it feels like a stroll through the park. In either case, using mindfulness meditation as a form of self-care helps you zoom out on your thoughts and build up your self-discipline muscles.

FOSTERING VAGINAL CONFIDENCE

Have you heard the saying that confidence comes from within? Well, it's true. You have the power to sexually and nonsexually affirm your body, particularly the parts that are hidden away—and sometimes used against us.

The messaging that you may be hearing from the outside world is that your pelvic parts should be hairless, perfectly shaped, and tight as a new jar of salsa. If that's how you like your vagina, that's great! If you feel self-conscious because your vagina doesn't look, smell, etc. like it "should," it's time to boost your confidence and practice mind-set work. "Mind-set" refers to the beliefs, values, and thoughts that collectively determine your state of being. Part of mind-set work for self-care down there involves actively resisting comparing yourself to your friends, family, models, and celebrities.... It's basically a full-time job. This is a lot harder than it sounds and requires careful curation of the voices and stories you let into your life, particularly before, during, and after sex.

Sacred Self-Care

Practice saying the following affirmation out loud or in your head: "My vagina is gorgeous and smells amazing." Your brain integrates that message every time you repeat it. So, even if you aren't feeling super-great about your vagina right now, you have the tools inside your very own mind to affirm and build vaginal confidence. Feeling great about yourself is an amazing benefit of self-care!

Part 4 Summary

In this part, you dove deeply into learning about the pleasure of sexuality. The act of sex can be one of the most intimate practices that your vagina and clitoris engage in. Yet, you may feel super-shy about it and don't really want to discuss it out loud. You also challenged yourself to think through your sexual practices. These are some self-care ideas to keep in mind:

- Figure out what fantasies and sex acts get you going, if any. To feel safe and sexy, you need to know what works for your body. Maybe you're not interested in sex at all. Or maybe you want to experience multiple orgasms a day. Either is amazing! Negotiating your sexuality can require a lot of self-exploration and sources of inspiration. At the same time, you must consider how social structures dictate the relations of power that privilege certain people's pleasure over others.
- Use lube, condoms, and sex toys that work for you. Just like any other hobby, sex can require some accessories. Different types of lube facilitate smooth entry. Various condoms protect against STIs for all sexes and genders. Vibrators, dildos, plugs, and more add some extra simulation and exploration. If you're planning to live lots of sexually active years, experimenting with body-safe adornments can keep things exciting and wet.

- Find space for sexual resilience in a messed-up modern world. The demands of patriarchy, capitalism, and colonialism may challenge your ability to find pleasure on a daily basis. You may feel like you barely have enough time to spend with your partners; maybe you are figuring out how to see yourself as a beautiful sexual being in an oppressive society. Amid this chaos, finding solitude, connection, and release will really benefit your well-being.

PART 5

The Modern-Day Vagina

Today's Vaginal Trends, Explained

Your elders left you rituals, medicines, and wisdom to get through your everyday life, care for your pelvic parts, and prepare for future generations to come. Today, you are facing challenges that your ancestors could never have dreamed of. You're dealing with water shortages, hyperconsumerism, toxin exposure, and overall environmental instability, all of which affect your vagina's (and your whole body's) capacity to have a safe place to call home.

In this part, you will explore vaginal care practices for surviving the twenty-first century. You'll discover self-care rituals that tell you how to take digital down time for down there, figure out how to bring your vagina on the road, and how to take care of your vagina in the workplace. You'll also see which vaginal trends to avoid or absorb. Even more, you'll explore the connection between gender equity, vaginal care, and being earth-friendly. Engaging in modern practices that give your pelvic parts nourishment, balance, and rest can help you not only survive but thrive in the world today.

UPLIFTING YOUR VAGINAL SELF-ESTEEM

Have you noticed how vaginas are often talked about as dirty, smelly, secret body parts? Companies feed off of these vaginal insecurities to make billions of dollars selling vaginal beautification products. It's true...societally, so much of the body image of people with vaginas is influenced by unrealistic standards created by advertisers who just want to make money. Vaginas in particular are portrayed as hairless, pimple-less, and always ready to have sex with a penis. Not to mention that every biology textbook shows the same image of what a vagina, ovaries, and uterus look like. With all this negative energy and erasure of diversity floating around, it can be difficult to practice positive self-care and have confidence in your vagina.

Sacred Self-Care

Take 20 minutes to digitally declutter. Go through your social media contacts and unfollow toxic accounts or any that make you feel bad about your vagina or yourself in general. Some might feel counterintuitive (like fitness and wellness accounts that are meant to be promoting "healthy" lifestyles). At the end, breathe a sigh of relief that you won't have to come across their newsfeeds anymore.

THINKING ABOUT
JADE EGGS

Today you can't go online without hearing about a new way to beautify or "improve" your already incredible vagina. You may have heard how jade eggs are now being sold as vaginal exercise balls. Basically, companies are claiming that you can make your vagina fit and toned by inserting a small green rock into it.

The mystery of how the jade egg practice originated remains unsolved. One study published in 2019 debunks jade eggs as an ancient Chinese practice. Researchers searched through pictures of five thousand–plus jade objects throughout various time periods in China, but didn't find a single mention of vaginal jade eggs in the archives. They concluded that vaginal egg manufacturers are just straight-up lying about the health benefits.

On the other hand, some pelvic weight lifters point out that many women and gender minorities struggle with pelvic floor dysfunction; they suggest that inserting jade eggs with strings attached into your vagina and then removing them can slowly build up pelvic muscle definition. However, many doctors disagree with this conclusion, so be sure to talk to your ob-gyn before trying this.

> **Sacred Self-Care**
>
> Write down a list of items to *avoid* sticking into your vagina for the purposes of tightening and/or self-care. If you are going to try a vaginal egg or another pelvic floor weight, run it by your doctor first.

TAKING CARE OF
PIERCINGS AND TATTOOS

Piercings and tattoos down there are a unique way to express yourself. Some people get a piercing to amplify their sexual experience or a tattoo to show off their personality in an intimate way. Whether you have a piercing and/or tattoo or are thinking about it getting one, it's important to remember that they require some cleaning and maintenance to keep them clean and infection-free.

Most body artists recommend that you shouldn't even think about getting a needle anywhere near down there until you accept that you'll need to spend some time every day over the next few weeks or months tending to your vagina, vulva, clitoris, or wherever you may pierce. Piercings and tattoos can get infected, itchy, too dry, too moist, and/or basically anything else that comes with broken skin. Your body artist will likely give you a rundown on how to keep the new part of you clean, so listen up and follow through. If you need more help, call your doctor. Be prepared to take on the challenge of protecting your precious parts—then enjoy the new addition to your body.

Sacred Self-Care

Practice self-care by letting your body heal completely before engaging in any kind of sex or activity that could irritate your piercing or tattoo. This includes playing with piercings or vigorously itching or picking at the area. Depending on your body's healing process, full healing may take anywhere from 6 weeks to 6 months. After that...enjoy the pleasure, and art!

PRACTICING PELVIC POLITICS

▼

Unfortunately, there is probably no other body part more regulated by politics than the vagina. Not surprisingly, the modern political system was built by and for cis men. Not many vaginas (cis women, trans men, nonbinary people, and more marginalized genders) sit in fancy chairs as heads of state across the world, but thankfully, those numbers are on the rise.

Lawmakers can choose to enact policies that support vaginal well-being, like providing free menstrual products in public bathrooms or making sure everyone has access to clean water. Or, they can control access to reproductive rights, like birth control or healthcare centers. When it comes to vaginal self-care, the politicians in your area and beyond actually have quite a lot of influence over the activities you can legally engage in.

Sacred Self-Care

Take ownership over your vagina—and practice self-care—by researching who to vote for in your next city, state, or province, and federal election. In most democratic places, you can easily find lists of candidates online. Newspaper and digital journalists do a lot of the work for you, showing comparisons of candidates and asking them for their opinions on such major topics as reproductive rights. Look for people whose views match yours and make sure to vote on Election Day.

UNDERSTANDING VAGINAL TOXIN EXPOSURE

The world you live in looks so different from what it looked like when your ancestors were practicing vaginal self-care. We've had some major wins and leaps forward, but, in terms of exposure to harmful substances, your vagina is in more danger than ever before. Chemicals in common household products can affect your health down there in all sorts of ways, from something relatively benign, like an itch, to serious illnesses, like cancer. Chemicals are present in many products you may use regularly, from tampons to talcum powder.

Now, the situation isn't as grim as it sounds—you probably have a healthy immune system, and your body has a built-in way to filter out toxins (thanks, liver!)—however, you never know when one more toxin is going to break the camel-toe's back, so you can't be too careful.

Sacred Self-Care

Start by reading these two lists: common toxins your vagina is exposed to every day and toxin-free choices. Over the next few months or even years, practice self-care by switching one or two toxic products you use to toxin-free versions (or even better, get rid of all your products with potentially harmful chemicals in them).

Toxic Products

- Scented pads, tampons, and liners
- Underwear washed with conventional, scented laundry soap
- Plastics in period products
- Synthetic hormones
- Douches and vaginal washes
- Talcum powder

Toxin-Free Choices

- Unscented period products
- Unscented laundry soap
- Plastic-free period products
- Natural methods of hormone balancing (Note: For people with PCOS, endometriosis, or for those who are taking gender-affirming hormones, dosing appropriately is usually more helpful than stopping completely. Ask your doctor and see the Resource List for more information.)
- Vagina allowed to self-clean
- Baking soda or cornstarch

TAKING YOUR VAGINA
TO WORK

Most likely, you are not free to bust out vulva massage oil in your office bathroom. But that doesn't mean you should ignore your vaginas during the 40-plus hours you're at work, either. First of all, be sure to take time off for important medical appointments—and don't feel bad about it, either. The patriarchal work world might not prioritize time off for vaginal health, but that doesn't mean you shouldn't be attentive to it. And when you are feeling the side effects of your period, such as cramps, at the office, bring a hot pack to put on your abdomen, drink lots of water, and take ibuprofen at regular intervals.

In addition to doing paid work, you probably also clean, cook, care for young ones and/or elders, and maintain friendships, all while trying to engage in self-care. Moreover, there are many warriors who push brand-new babies out of our vaginas and bodies. Practice self-care by prioritizing time for you and asking for help when you need it. You are important; you and your vagina deserve to take the time to ensure your pelvic health.

Sacred Self-Care

One small change you can make today is to download and use a free work timer application like Be Focused or focus booster. These apps give you reminders to take breaks to use the bathroom, drink water, tend to your period, or do some stretches for your pelvis. You can customize the timing of your reminders to suit your lifestyle and personal needs.

SUPPORTING YOUR VAGINA IN THE DIGITAL WORLD

The average person spends about 5 hours of the day looking at a screen. While the Internet has abundant benefits, it can also hurt your pelvic health.

After all, when you're looking at screens, you're usually sitting down, slumped over, with your neck, wrists, and backside in awkward positions for long periods of time. Maybe you struggle to keep your feet on the floor and tend to stay in one place for hours on end. This position can increase pelvic pain. Thankfully, there are easy adjustments you can to do to make sure your pelvis is happy and healthy for many years to come.

Sacred Self-Care

For pelvic self-care, make sure to add at least 5 minutes of pelvic stretches into your day. Spend some of your sitting-down time researching stretches on the Internet. My favorite stretches include examples from the Egoscue Clinic in Austin, Texas, and Geethanjali Yoga in Pondicherry, India. Both have videos up on *YouTube*. Next, be sure you're sitting in the right position for pelvic health when doing the following steps.

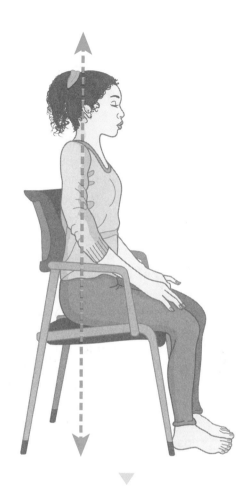

Create a space that allows you to sit comfortably in a chair and be mindful of your pelvic wellness. Keep your feet flat on the floor, about hip-width apart, and sit in a position where your hips are slightly higher than your knees. This is a game changer. Keep your weight evenly distributed on your pelvis and try not to cross your legs. Be sure to keep your back and neck straight and your shoulders pulled back, so they remain aligned with your hips. This position keeps the pressure off of your pelvic floor and is a great way to let self-care down there change your life.

TAKING YOUR VAGINA
ON THE ROAD

Whether you love traveling or are more of a homebody, everyone has to head out of town sometime or another. Maybe you love the excitement of leaving home and exploring new places, and do it frequently, but even people who don't travel much are summoned to an out-of-town wedding or work conference once in a while. With travel becoming easier and faster in this modern world, it's important to think about your vaginal and pelvic health just like you do your suitcase or carry-on.

Traveling is actually very difficult on your pelvic region. From getting sand in your vagina to enduring a long, bumpy bus ride, to sitting in one position for ages, you might find yourself sore or achy if you don't think ahead. Plus, traveling can shake up your routine and change your access to basic necessities. (For example, your destination might not have the period products your body is used to.) Don't worry, though—being prepared for travel will help your trip go smoothly.

Sacred Self-Care

Spend an evening filling a travel-sized cosmetic bag with key items from your pelvic self-care pantry (see the Creating a Pelvic Self-Care Pantry entry in Part 2). Be sure to include essentials like:

- Medicines
- Period products

- Fun snacks
- Contact information for your preferred healthcare provider (you can add this to your phone)

To keep you feeling grounded on your trip, add a special little item, like:

- Stone
- Crystal
- Totem

When you are rushing to the bus, car, train, or plane, you can feel assured that you've taken all the steps necessary to have a smooth journey.

BEING PREPARED
ON-THE-GO

Traveling can offer unique opportunities for sexy scheming—whether with your partner or with somebody you meet at your destination. Away from home, it can be easier to let go of all your sexual hang-ups and put yourself out there. Still, whether you're around the corner or across the globe, it's important to communicate with potential partners about your relationship status, boundaries, and expectations. Being prepared mentally, physically, and spiritually will help make the experience memorable for all the right reasons. Keep your vagina, cervix, and whole pelvis out of harm's way by knowing the sex laws of the place you are visiting and finding a private space to get down and dirty.

Sacred Self-Care

Add condoms (male, female, or both) to your list of things to pack. If you are going to be having intercourse (penis meeting vagina), keep an emergency contraception pill in your luggage for those moments where everything else fails or you are in an unexpected situation. You should be mindful that emergency contraception is illegal in some countries. There is no greater post-orgasm letdown than dealing with the consequences of a broken condom. And there is no greater kind of self-care than being sure that you're the one in control of your sexual health.

CHOOSING AFFIRMING SWIMWEAR

When it's time to wear a swimsuit, even the most secure people with vaginas can quickly revert to judging themselves against impossible beauty standards. Maybe you find that magazine articles about beach bodies and ads with lingerie models seem to materialize as soon as someone says, "There's going to be a pool!"

Whether you are sporting a 10-year-old bikini or this season's burkini, know that you and your vagina look fabulous in it. Even better than making you look cute, wearing a swimsuit means spending time in the water. The gentle movement and flow of water can soothe pelvic pain, cool you off during PMS, and allow you to connect with something bigger than yourself—water, the ultimate giver of life.

Sacred Self-Care

Take an afternoon off to shop in person or online for swimwear that makes you feel amazing in your body. You can find bathing suit brands to fit any budget, style, and size, but whatever suit you choose, be sure to buy a suit with a cut and fabric that doesn't rub painfully against your underwear line. Moreover, make sure to remove your swimsuit and let it dry as soon as possible after getting out of the water. Hanging out in a damp swimsuit can create excess moisture down there, which can lead to pelvic skin issues and/or infections.

FINDING VAGINAL RESOURCES ANYWHERE, ANYTIME

Did you know that there is a version of *Wikipedia* just for your vagina and pelvic area? *Gynopedia* (https://gynopedia .org) is a nonprofit website that provides vaginal care options for people traveling all over the globe. With just a few clicks and scrolls on your smartphone, you can find a vaginal care clinic in countries from Argentina to Zimbabwe—plus key information about local laws, availability of contraceptives, and more.

The digital index is user-generated and broken down by country and city. While the options are pretty heteronorma-tive and focus on preventing pregnancy, the crowdsourced information is still super-valuable when you are in an unfamil-iar place. If you notice a random new red patch on your pelvis or experience spotting during your menstrual cycle while on the road, turn to this site for help—and know that you are not alone in these experiences. We've all been there at one time or another.

Sacred Self-Care

Practice self-care by asking yourself how your vaginal and pelvic symptoms feel on a scale of 1 to 10. Based on your self-assessment, you can decide which action to take next. You might want to do a light vaginal steam in your hotel room, go immediately to the clos-est medical doctor (which you can find on the *Gynopedia* website), or make a phone call to one of your preferred healthcare providers and ask for their advice.

HEALING FROM
TRAUMA

Many people with vaginas will experience little *t* or big *T* trauma in their lives. Little *t* trauma can include things like microaggressions (e.g. a sexist comment made by a coworker) or accidentally pulling your tampon out too quickly (ouch!). Big *T* trauma can include life-changing events like sexual assault, domestic violence, birth trauma, breakups, accidents, losses, depression, and eating disorders. Layered on top of individual encounters are the ongoing impacts of colonialism, patriarchy, and capitalism, which may make you feel like your pelvic area isn't under your own control. When traumas involve your pelvic area, your life-force energy can be destabilized.

While it may seem grim, there can also be beauty in being aware of your traumas down there. Research shows that talking about a particularly hurtful incident can release 50 percent of the stress associated with it. It is well known that stress affects your pelvic processes (such as your body's ability to ovulate), so releasing that stress or trauma is especially beneficial for pelvic self-care. Acknowledging and beginning (or continuing on) the journey of healing from trauma makes you more resilient, develops your own unique perspective on the world, and strengthens your ability to set boundaries that help you feel safe.

Sacred Self-Care

Practice self-care by making an appointment with a therapist or counselor who focuses on body-based therapeutic practices in your area. If you're searching online, search for key words like somatic therapy, art therapy, or energy healing. Look for a therapist whose values align with yours and who makes you feel heard. Sometimes all you need is one or two sessions to kickstart your journey toward healing your pelvic trauma. Keep in mind that some therapists offer free initial consultations.

MEDITATING ON YOUR YONI

We live an incredibly fast-paced life, packing a ton of commuting, balancing, speed-eating, and screen time into one day. Believe it or not, when your brain goes into overdrive, your vagina can feel it too. You might have a hard time focusing during sex or rush through a shower or pelvic stretches. When it comes to self-care down there, it's never been more important to slow down, breathe, and be in the present.

Mindfulness meditation can help with this. It is a practice that is reminiscent of prayer and ceremony from many spiritual faiths, although it's now used in a fairly secular way. For vaginal self-care, mindfulness meditation can involve sitting in silence while breathing slowly and concentrating on your vagina. Meditation also raises awareness of your thought patterns—you will start to notice which thoughts come up again and again as you try to quiet your mind. This knowledge can help you address negative or harmful ideas you might have about your pelvic region.

Sacred Self-Care

Get into a comfortable, still position. Start by tuning into the natural rhythm of your breath. Then, see if you can send the air all the way down to your pelvis with each inhale. After some breaths, begin to notice what images, ideas, and memories are coming up for you. Try picturing yourself on a bridge, with your thoughts flowing like a river under you without judgment. Let the river simply flow underneath while you focus on being on the bridge and breathing.

PRIORITIZING VAGINAL SELF-CARE EVERY DAY

The world is a busy place for a pelvis. You might be hustling in work or school, raising a family, taking care of pets, maintaining friendships and relationships, learning new skills, caring for elders, or some combination of these—all while maybe growing a baby or having your period. Oh, and did you find time to sleep?

With this harried lifestyle, building in a pelvic "self-care down there" practice every day becomes incredibly necessary. Yet, it can feel like the hardest thing to make time for. You might ask, "Why do I need to take time for my pelvis? I barely have time to eat lunch!" Remember, the pelvis, or root chakra, is an energy center that can get out of balance if its basic physical, mental, emotional, and spiritual needs are not met. If you're still not sure it's worth your precious time, imagine building a house. You'd want to set a solid foundation in place before you build upward, right? Don't forget to tend to your physical base as well.

Sacred Self-Care

Build in a practice of forgiveness. Forgive yourself daily for all the moments when you did something you wish you hadn't because you felt frustrated, irritable, angry, and/or just needed a nap. Sending breath down to your root chakra can provide a source of strength during these moments. Your inner self is telling you something through these emotions and physical signs. So, listening to your body and mind can promote vaginal well-being and an overall sense of harmony among your body, mind, and spirit.

MAKING PROACTIVE PELVIC DECISIONS

You face decision after decision every day about your vagina. Which underwear should you put on? What activities should you do based on your menstrual cycle? Should you invest in a new vibrator? What does the doctor mean when they say you need a pap smear? What birth control method should you use? The list of questions is endless and can feel overwhelming.

With the Internet at your fingertips, it's easy to get lost in an online rabbit hole and come out feeling like you have to rethink your approach to vaginal health...and maybe your entire life. If that happens to you, stop, breathe, and recenter yourself before you take any action. Remember that you and you alone are in charge of making decisions about your pelvic health. Don't let anyone pressure you to do something you don't want to do. Be proactive and knowledgeable about your choices. Always make decisions in a mind-set of self-care.

Sacred Self-Care

If you find yourself in a situation where you don't know what to do, take a few minutes to write down all the trusted resources and knowledgeable people you have in your toolkit. If you can't think of any resources for a particular area, check out the Resource List at the end of this book. Know that most vaginal or pelvic imbalances take a least a day or two (if not months) to get back into sync, so try to be patient. Moreover, in these moments of uncertainty, know that no one else knows your body better than you do.

Part 5 Summary

In this part, you explored, questioned, and tested out some modern trends and discoveries for self-care down there. These necessary self-care tips, which range in topic from politics to jade eggs, focus on helping you manage your pelvic wellness in the twenty-first century. Some self-care ideas to keep in mind include the following:

- Fight back against exposure to toxins. Skip over the body products that have toxins in them, like scented laundry soaps and scented period products, and switch to toxin-free versions. Moreover, put up boundaries between yourself and social toxins, like nasty politicians, social media accounts that make you feel bad about yourself, or unhealthy relationships. Taking action against toxic materials or beings supports your pelvic wellness.
- Try out pelvic health prevention strategies, which help you build your capacity to bounce back when something is going on down there. You learned how to practice forgiveness, meditation, and seek counsel from mentors, healers, and friends.
- Engage in self-awareness. Many of the self-care tips in this part aim to help you increase your knowledge of yourself, your body, and the environment around you. You can make connections between your pelvic wellness, the thoughts you

have about your vagina, and/or the social context you live in. By raising your consciousness or "getting woke," you support pelvic health for people with vaginas around the world.

RESOURCE LIST

These are recommended resources. As always...what happens with your body is your choice, so feel free to really get into the resources that you align with and let go of the ones that don't.

Centre for Menstrual Cycle and Ovulation Research

www.cemcor.org

Up-to-date scientific evidence on menstrual cycles, PCOS, ovulation, fibroids, pelvic bone health, and more from a feminist endocrinologist and team.

Clue Period & Cycle Tracker App

https://helloclue.com

Clue is a vaginal care app and website that delivers essential education about health, periods, and sex. It is one of the few vaginal and sexual health websites that use nonbinary, nonhetero language to talk about sex, gender, and sexuality.

Fertility Friday

https://fertilityfriday.com

Podcast, video, and blog posts about the fertility awareness method of natural birth control.

Free Do-It-Yourself Vaginal Steam Tutorial by Steamy Chick

www.steamychick.com/diy

Free step-by-step tutorial on how to perform a vaginal steam in your home.

Handbook of International Centers for Survivors of Sexual Assault and Harassment

https://headington-institute.org/files/international_centers_for_survivors_of_sexual_assault_45553.pdf

A directory of clinics and care centers for people all over the world who are survivors of sexual assault and their allies.

The Heavy Flow Podcast

http://amandalaird.ca/the-heavy-flow-podcast/

Intersectional and diverse interviews from leaders in the vaginal and menstrual health movement.

Hygiene and You *YouTube* Channel

www.youtube.com/playlist?list=PLdn87RYhFrpAO3TZXQD6wHK8DDGykJc4f

Videos on vaginal health topics ranging from how to measure cervix length to PCOS.

IM With Periods Nerd Zone

https://imwithperiods.com/nerd-zone

This section of the *IM With Periods* website offers a longer, comprehensive list of resources for all things related to vaginal health and wellness.

MakeLoveNotPorn

http://makelovenotporn.com

MakeLoveNotPorn is pro-sex. Pro-porn. Pro-knowing the difference. It is the world's first user-generated, human-curated, social sex video-sharing platform.

ACKNOWLEDGMENTS

The universe, cosmos, and spirits are tricksters. They work in very mysterious ways. *Self-Care Down There* is in your hands because of a little bit of magic as well as the work of many amazing people who made this book a reality.

My bhanjis at *Blume* (www.blume.com) are bringing toxin-free period products, and soon sex education, to folks. They agreed to do a skill share with me for their blog so I could start to publicly test out my perspectives of vaginas, periods, and the modern world. Cate Prato, one of my amazing editors at Adams Media, read the post and pitched the idea of *Self-Care Down There* to me. Just months later, we sealed the deal and had a manuscript in place. The whole team at Adams Media, especially Cate Prato, Katie Corcoran Lytle, and Sarah Armour, who have made magic into reality through their dedicated production and promotion of the book.

I couldn't have made it through the writing process alive without the enormous support of my writing and research kin. Shruti Buddhavarapu, my collaborator and social justice editor, continues to push me to always redesign our inclusive, intersectional thinking. Dr. Jerilynn Prior and the CeMCOR team remind me to be vigilant in our pursuits for research and practice. The counter-narrative must go on.

All the volunteers, staff, and community members at the Vancouver Women's Health Collective keep me grounded circa 2014. My peers, colleagues, teachers, and mentors at the University of British Columbia, York University, and Dalhousie University poke our heads up every once in a while to chat as we make our marks in the nebulous, confusing, and weird space of academia. Cheers to my fellow nerds and members of the Society for Menstrual Cycle Research. May we wear menstrual cups, sea sponges, cloths, and conference badges until the end. I'm forever in solidarity with all the therapists, healers, nurses, doctors, and more who share their wisdom about our bodies, minds, and spirits, especially my fertility awareness method teacher, Lisa Hendrickson-Jack of *Fertility Friday*.

I have to give it up to all the productivity podcasters out there who fueled my motivation tank. To my business coach, Dielle, who is carving a path to follow in the jungle of online entrepreneurship. To Meenu for cheering me on and keeping me accountable to my goals and self-care. To Melanie for taking part in IM With Periods social media and spreading the word even further. To my friends and allies everywhere who show endless excitement and keep my imposter syndrome in check. Namely, Alysha, Megan, Leanna, Emily Wei-Hsin, Midori, Guida, Hera, and Carla, who get me out for power walks, tea dates, and dance parties.

A special thanks goes to my family and housemates (including the furry ones) who have put up with my endless rants about periods and vaginas for the last few years. Thanks for going on *YouTube* spirals with me, trying to figure out the Punjabi word for "ovulation." As for my relatives who come across this book unexpectedly—surprise!

Finally, my partner, Jeff, deserves boundless gratitude for remaining patient during every freak-out, every new idea, every dessert run, every painful period, and more.

INDEX

ABOUT THE AUTHOR

Taq Kaur Bhandal is a researcher, writer, menstrual health coach, dog lady, and the founder and CEO of IM With Periods. She curates the company *Instagram* account @imwithperiods to share knowledge of periods and cycles for all menstruators and has blogged for *Blume*, a website for safe, sustainable period products for women and girls. Taq is currently working toward a PhD at the University of British Columbia Social Justice Institute and is a member of the Society for Menstrual Cycle Research.